Additional Praise for

365 Health and
Happiness Boosters

"M.J. Ryan proves it again—this time better than ever: the brief, simple, and genial way to self-improvement is the most effective. You'll treasure this practical guide to building the happiness habit, one enjoyable day after another—especially if your 'happiness quotient' needs a boost."

> —David Kundtz, author of *Everyday Serenity*

"My heart lifted as I held this little book full of wisdom and positive insights. The book allows you to gently reflect on the good things in your life and set your sails, with greater confidence, for the new shores you wish to explore."

> —Mary Ellen, author of *Expect Miracles*

"By giving us daily happiness activities that touch our hearts and souls, M.J. Ryan empowers each of us to experience the joy of living and, ultimately, the joy of being alive, no matter what."

> —Jackie Waldman, author of *The Courage to Give*
> and *Teens with the Courage to Give*

365

Health
and Happiness
Boosters

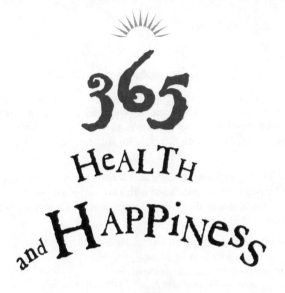

365
HeALTh
and HAPPiNess
BOOSTers

M. J. Ryan

CONARI PRESS
Berkeley, California

Conari Press books are distributed by Publishers Group West.
Cover art direction: Ame Beanland
Cover and book design: Claudia Smelser
Cover illustrations: Nicholas Wilton and Claudia Smelser
Interior illustration: Joan Carroll

Library of Congress Cataloging-in-Publication Data

Ryan. M. J. (Mary Jane)
    365 health and happiness boosters / M. J. Ryan
      p.   cm.
    ISBN: 1-57324-500-3
    1. Happiness—Problems, exercises, etc. I. Title: three hundred sixty-five health and happiness boosters. II. Title: three hundred sixty-five health and happiness boosters. III. Title.
BF575.H27 .R93 2000
I58—dc21   99–088973

Printed in the United States of America on recycled paper

00 01 02 03 DATA 10 9 8 7 6 5 4 3 2 1

Life is short and it's up to you
to make it sweet.

Sadie Delany,
coauthor of *Having Our Say*

A Little Course in Happiness

What we nurture in ourselves will grow;
that is nature's eternal law.
—Anonymous

Happiness, the sheer joy of being alive, is something we all long to experience. Indeed, it is such an important shared value that the Declaration of Independence identifies it as one of only three unalienable rights: life, liberty, and the pursuit of happiness.

I'm relatively new to the pursuit of happiness. Or rather, I may have pursued it all my life, but only recently have I begun to *experience* it on anything that could be considered a consistent basis. That's because, like so many of us, I wasn't taught how to be happy. In fact, like most of us, I was misinformed as to where happiness lies. I was led to believe that some people were born happy and others were not, and there wasn't anything you could do about that. I was taught that happiness came from doing well in school, having the right job, the perfect mate, the dream house, the $30,000 BMW. I was taught to focus on all that was wrong in my life, all the ways I had been victimized and abused, instead of paying attention to what was working, what was right about me. I was trained in "if onlys"— if only my mate would come home from work earlier I'd be happy; if only I made $20,000 more a year I'd be happy; if only I didn't have to work I'd be happy. I spent my time trying to make my "if onlys" come true and complained bitterly if they did not.

Then one day I decided that I was sick and tired of being depressed, negative, and miserable, and I went on a campaign to learn how to be happy. You're holding the results of my ten years of learning. It contains all I know—from the completely frivolous to the profound—about being happy. I offer it in the hope that it will help the practice of happiness to spread.

Because I'm not alone. According to research, about two-thirds of us don't know how to be happy. In 1957, in the United States, a study was done in which people were asked whether they were happy with what they had in life. Around 30 percent said yes. The study was repeated in 1992 and the same percentage said yes, despite the fact that the standard of living had increased dramatically in that time. What this shows, besides that possessions can't make us happy, is that about one-third of the population knows the secret to happiness—that it is an inside job, and is not contingent on possessions, status, or even life circumstances. Whether from inherited temperament, early childhood training, or conscious cultivation, those people are happy. Fortunately the rest of us can learn.

That is the assumption behind this book—that *you*

can be happier, no matter who you are or what challenges you face. A great deal of how to be happier has to do with changing your outlook, but it also has to do with what you eat, how you interact with others, even how well you sleep.

Most of the other books on happiness are some person's theory of what you need to do to become happy. This book is different. Rather than theory, it offers 365 concrete things you can do, just for today, to experience happiness. The reason I've structured it this way is that I believe that we need to experience happiness on a daily basis, rather than just as "peak moments" on special occasions—our wedding, a trip to an exotic place, the birth of a child. Indeed, research confirms that the best path to happiness is a daily one. As Edward Diener, a University of Illinois researcher specializing in happiness, said recently in the *Santa Barbara News-Press*, "Happiness is how frequently you're happy, not how intensely."

Hence the daily format. Some of my suggestions involve attitudes that we can change to create more happiness overall in our lives; others are concrete things we can do to lift our spirits in the moment; still others are environmental changes or nutritional supplements we can try. Some are lighthearted, others quite serious. All will have positive effects on our minds, bodies, and spirits. That's because our minds and bodies are not really separate, and as science has begun to demonstrate, experiencing positive emotions such as happiness strengthens the immune systems, which enables the body to resist disease and recover more quickly from illness, through the release of endorphins and other compounds into the bloodstream. Not only are endorphins the body's natural painkillers, they also stimulate dilation of the blood vessels, which leads to a relaxed heart.

Conversely, negative emotions, such as worry, anger, and fear, reduce the number and slow the movement of disease-fighting white cells in the bloodstream, and contribute to the development of stroke and heart disease by dumping high levels of adrenaline into the blood. Adrenaline constricts blood vessels, particularly to the heart, raising blood pressure and potentially damaging arteries and the heart itself.

In a landmark overview study, Howard Friedman and S. Boothby-Kewley analyzed 101 studies of the relationship between mood and disease. They found that people with a predominance of negative emotions were twice as likely to get sick as those who had more positive attitudes. In fact, they found that chronic negative emotions were as big a risk factor in developing disease as smoking and high cholesterol. So the more we can cultivate happiness, the healthier we're likely to be!

All my suggestions are things that can be done right now, in this moment or at least in the course of a normal, hectic day. (I hate those books with unrealistic ideas—ones that are too hard to do, too complicated, or too much to tackle; who has time to track *anything* for a month?) You can use the book in one of three ways. Each suggestion is dated, so you can follow one a day throughout the year. Or you can just open a page at random and do what appeals to you. Or you can use the index in the back to pursue certain issues: methods for sleeping better, for instance, or dealing with fear if that is blocking your happiness. I call it "a course in happiness," because if you even do an eighth of these 365 suggestions, you will learn how to be happy.

Many of us think of the pursuit of happiness as a selfish one, that to choose to be as happy as possible will mean that we won't care about the world or its problems. Of course, the opposite tends to be true. As proof, all you have to do is answer the question that Dennis Prager asks in his book *Happiness Is a Serious Problem:* "Do you feel more positively disposed toward other people and do you want to treat other people better when you are happy or when you are unhappy?"

That's the most wonderful thing about practicing happiness—it will come back to us tenfold. For our happiness ripples out into the world, creating even more. As Barry Neil Kaufman says, "If just one of us changes our beliefs and teaches happiness and love, then that attitude or information goes out into the connective tissue of the community and enhances the aptitude for happiness of the entire human group." So not only are we learning to be happy for ourselves, but for our families, our friends, our work groups and neighborhoods, and the world as a whole.

May happiness continue to grow in ourselves and in the world.

What Matters to You?

The great political and spiritual leader Mahatma Gandhi once said, "Happiness is when what you think, what you say, and what you do are in harmony." On this first day of the new year, it's a good time to take the opportunity to look at your values. What is most important to you? Do you express those values in how you live?

When I ask myself those questions, I realize that kindness and gratitude are very important to me, but I don't express them as much as I would like. Today I make a commitment to myself to practice gratitude by saying a blessing before dinner, and to look for occasions to be more kind to others.

What about you? The deep sense of joy that comes from living our values is a priceless gift.

Mark Your Calendars

I always love the beginning of the year when I get a new planner and transfer over all my phone numbers, birthdays, and upcoming meetings. I guess it's the sense of starting fresh in a brand-new year.

This year, as you mark your calendar with the dates you need to remember, pick at random four, just four, days and put a special symbol on those days—a star, a smiley face, whatever. Then, when you come to them during the year, give yourself a treat.

This will bring you fivefold happiness: the four treats and the smile it brings now in anticipation of what's to come.

Pray for Happiness

Prayer works, so why not use it on behalf of our happiness? There have been many studies done recently on the efficacy of prayer. The one that impressed me the most was done on 393 heart attack patients; 192 were prayed for without their knowing it; the rest were not. All other treatment was exactly the same. Of the group that was prayed for, there were fewer fatalities and more rapid recoveries.

So pray for happiness. And be sure to ask directly— we usually want what we want because we think it will make us happy, but we forget to ask for happiness directly. Today, ask for whatever will make you happy, without assuming you know what that is.

Understand What Happiness Is

We all want more happiness—but do we even know what it is? Happiness is a feeling we experience in our bodies. In that way, it is always self-generated—we experience it internally. But many of us think of happiness as a feeling of pleasure based on some external happening—we got the raise we wanted, we just ate a fabulous meal. But true happiness isn't contingent on circumstances. It is a sense of contentment that exists independently of the good fortune that might find us. Proof of that comes from a study of lottery winners. Just six months after winning, they report they are no happier than they were before their windfalls.

We find true happiness from a sense of contentment that we experience when we let go of our judgments and accept ourselves, other people, and life as it is, no matter how imperfect. Try it just for today. When you notice yourself judging someone or something as bad (the screaming baby, the insensitive coworker, your own frustration), pause, take a breath, and say to yourself, "They are (or I am) doing the best that they can." At the end of the day, notice whether acceptance has brought you more peace and contentment. Remember, as Leonard Sweet says in *A Cup of Coffee at the Soul Café*, "Our duty is not to see through one another, but to see one another through."

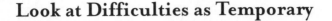

Look at Difficulties as Temporary

Research on optimists and pessimists has uncovered the fact that pessimists believe that whatever bad thing is happening is immutable, while optimists view the same thing as only temporary.

Boy, does that ring true for me, the reformed pessimist. When I was in my early twenties, I hurt my back and spent over a year in bed. Finally I went to a pain center, where I learned a variety of things. Perhaps the most useful was to rank my pain from one to ten every day, with one being mild discomfort and ten agony. Why was it so helpful? Because I understood that it changed. Before that, I would say it hurt the same every day; once I began numbering, I saw that some days were eights, but others were fives. Sometimes I hurt more, but other times less. I remember the day I thought to myself, if it can go down, maybe it can go away, at least for a little while. And by changing my thinking about my problem—believing that it could get better—eventually it did. I still experience pain, but my relationship to it is completely transformed.

What in your life could benefit from a reframing as only being temporary? A job you don't like? A problem with someone in your life? Feeling stuck is what causes most of the misery.

Use Good Scents

Smells can be mood elevators. Here are some ways to bring good scents into your day:

Light a candle with a favorite scent before you go to bed. It will perfume the room. My favorite is Casablanca lily. Jasmine is a good choice too—it induces optimism. Just be sure to blow out the candle before you fall asleep.

Apply a scented lotion or one or two drops of your favorite essential oil to your temples and rub gently. Various body stores even have specialized "pulse point" lotions.

I Will Believe in You
Every Day of My Life

I have a wonderful friend named Molly Fumia who is one of the best happiness boosters I have ever met. Being with her is like being wrapped in a cocoon of unconditional love and support.

Recently I opened a package from her, and a little two by two-inch card (probably made on her computer) fell out. It read, "I will believe in you every day of my life"— Elliot to E.T. from the movie *E.T.* My heart soared. What a fabulous message—I felt instantly uplifted. And if it cheered me, who has a healthy dose of self-esteem, imagine what it can do for someone in great need of support and encouragement!

Who in your life needs to hear such a message? You? Your spouse? Your children? Spread some joy around— send an e-mail, write, or call someone and tell them, "I will believe in you every day of my life" and see how you—and they—feel.

Pick Up the Eggs

Buddhists have wonderful teaching stories. This is one told about Aachan Cha, a Thai monk and teacher. A monk at his monastery kept complaining to him about all the other monks—they should be better meditators, they should eat less. Finally Aachan Cha turned to him and said, "You are like somebody who keeps chickens and then goes out in the morning and picks up the droppings instead of the eggs."

What eggs are you ignoring right now because you're so focused on the droppings?

Make a Worry List

I am a world-class worrier by habit, and it definitely gets in the way of my being happy. So over the years I've had to learn various "anti-worrying" techniques, so that all my mental energy doesn't go into worrying. Here's two things that are incredibly simple yet effective:

Sometimes just writing down what is bothering you can be tremendously effective in letting it go. Write down in list form, one after another, all the things that are bothering you. It really helps to see them on paper—they are now outside of you rather than internalized, and they can be approached one at a time rather than seeming like an overwhelming mishmash.

Rating your worries on a scale of one to ten, with ten being the absolute worst thing that could happen—the death of your child or your mate, for example—is also very effective. When you make ten so extreme, it's easier to keep some perspective on the everyday worries you might be experiencing. An annoying boss? A project that needs finishing in short order? Clearly not a ten.

Have a Tuna Fish Sandwich

Regularly eating tuna, salmon, and other fish high in Omega-3 fatty acids relieves depression, according to studies done by the National Institutes of Health (NIH). The reason? They increase levels of serotonin in the blood, which helps to increase calm and a sense of well-being. "The brain is essentially made of fat," explains Dr. Joseph Hibbeln of the NIH. "Some of the fats that are necessary for proper brain functioning cannot be manufactured by the body. They must be obtained in the diet."

In the past, notes Hibbeln, humans ate foods rich in these oils. Now we don't, and depression and other mental illnesses are on the rise. If fish isn't your thing, flaxseed and canola oil also raise serotonin levels, and fish-oil supplements can be purchased at nutrition centers or health food stores.

Fake It

Wisdom comes from all kinds of places. I was reading *Vanity Fair* recently (a guilty pleasure), and came across an interview with Jordan's Queen Noor about life after the death of her beloved husband, King Hussein. She said of him, "He always felt his responsibility was to project only the most positive, constructive, caring, loving, comforting spirit to everyone he encountered, no matter what he was feeling inside. It was easy to see that that was one way of giving the best of oneself to others, and also it happens to be a very peaceful way to live your life—to whatever extent you can do it."

Research confirms the wisdom of the king's technique. Researchers David Myers and Edward Diener have discovered that if you "fake" a trait of happy people, you will begin to feel happier too. For example, subjects who pretended to have high self-esteem began to feel as if they did, and those who were asked to smile actually felt happier.

Rejoice in Love

Love—the love of friends and family—is a precious gift that is often unacknowledged when we get caught up in our expectations and judgments or the just plain busyness of our day. But isn't the mere fact that you are loved by those who care about you amazing? After all, you aren't perfect; you have your own foibles (as Paul Pearsall said in a recent speech, "Raise your hand if you would like to be married to you"); yet those who love you love you regardless of your flaws.

Isn't that love worth celebrating right now?

Create a Morning Wonder Ritual

The great musician Pablo Casals once said, "For the past eighty years, I have started each day in the same manner. It is not a mechanical routine but something essential to my daily life. I go to the piano and I play two preludes and fugues of Bach. I cannot think of doing otherwise. It is a sort of benediction on the house. But that is not its only meaning for me. It is a rediscovery of the world in which I have the joy of being a part. It fills me with awareness of the wonder of life, with a feeling of the incredible marvel of being a human being."

What small thing can you do when you wake up in the morning to tap into that sense of marvel before you start your day? Play a special piece of music? Read something inspirational? For me, it's cuddling in bed with my daughter, looking up at the redwood tree framed in the skylight, and listening to the birds sing.

Stand Up Straight

I know I probably sound like your mother, but motivational speakers Drs. Michael Mercer and Maryann Troiani, authors of *Spontaneous Optimism*, claim that if you learn to keep your head up, shoulders back, and chest out, you'll feel better. "Before you can straighten up your head, you first need to straighten up your body," they maintain. "When you slouch, your mood takes somewhat of a dive. When you notice that, immediately straighten up. That is your first step to boost your mood." Try it today.

Reach across Difference

Today is the birthday of Dr. Martin Luther King, Jr. He was full of all kinds of wisdom. One of my most favorite sayings of his is, "We may have all come on different ships, but we're in the same boat now." We are all, everyone of us, in the same boat, but we have a tendency to cluster together with people just like ourselves. It makes us feel comfortable, safe. But it can also cause us to stagnate, to miss out on the happiness that comes from different perspectives.

So, in honor of Dr. King's birthday, how about reaching out to someone who is different in some way from you? Someone of a different race, sexual orientation, culture, age? Ask a coworker you've ignored to lunch; invite your deaf neighbors to dinner. Stretch yourself and enjoy the feeling that comes from reaching out.

Have Hope

Sometimes life can be so difficult that the only happiness we can find is through hope. Hope is an important spiritual discipline, the ballast that keeps us going even as we seem to be sinking. "Hope is a state of mind," writes Vaclav Havel, "not of the world. . . . It is a dimension of the soul and it's not dependent on some observation of the world or estimate of the situation. . . . Hope is definitely not the same thing as optimism. It is not the conviction that something will turn out well, but the certainty that something makes sense, regardless of how it turns out."

If you're low on hope, try this meditation by Sue Patton Thoele: "Gently close your eyes and focus on your breath. . . . With each inhalation, imagine that you are drawing in the energy of hope into your body. It doesn't matter if you feel hopeful, the intention toward hopefulness is enough for now. Briefly think of any circumstance, feeling, or belief that is creating stormy seas for you. Notice that a short distance away is a quiet, serene, and welcoming harbor. Angels, friends, or other emissaries beckon for you to come into the harbor. . . . As you enter the harbor of hope, you are greeted by Beings who will care for you compassionately. Rest with them and allow them to minister to you."

Combat Delight Deficiency Disorder

Delight Deficiency Disorder is a condition identified by Paul Pearsall, author of *The Pleasure Prescription,* that results in anger, irritability, aggression, and impatience. "When you're not getting delight in your daily diet, your body begins to starve for its spiritual nutrients." Its cause? Taking ourselves too seriously, trying to control what can't be controlled, forgetting to indulge in the simple pleasures of life. The cure? Lighten up and laugh, realize that we can control very little, and find healthy ways to bring pleasure back into your life. "If you don't find a balance between pressure and pleasure, your epitaph is going to read, 'Got everything done, died anyway.'"

In many ways, this whole book is conceived of as a antidote to Delight Deficiency Disorder, and you will read about many ways to bring happiness and pleasure back into your life. For today, just ask yourself, "In what ways am I suffering from DDD? When was the last time I really laughed? Do I find myself chronically impatient with people?" Awareness alone will bring a bit of relief from this disease.

Send a Note of Appreciation
Out of the Blue

As an editor, I have worked with many authors. Some become friends; others remain more at a distance. I recently got a letter from a person who fell into the latter category. We'd worked together pleasantly, and that was that. Then, years later, this letter. In it, he said that he just realized recently how much I had taught him about writing and wanted to thank me. What a wonderful surprise! It was the nicest thing that had happened to me in a long time. And we both got to be happy—me when I got the letter, him while writing it and when I later called to thank him for a wonderful gesture.

Call or write someone who did something nice for you in the past and thank them. You'll feel great.

Get Connected

If you want to share happiness with others, check out the Secret Society of Happy People at **www.sohp.com**. The society was formed "to encourage people to talk more about happy events and moments and discourage the social backlash that often accompanies this.

"Somewhere between *The Ed Sullivan Show* and *The Jerry Springer Show*, talking about being happy became politically incorrect. We're more comfortable airing our dirty laundry than telling people [we've] had a great moment.

"We believe happiness is contagious and that when more people talk about happy events and moments it will be comfortable for everyone to do it. Eventually the language of happiness will again be part of everyday conversation." Check it out.

Reframe Mistakes

The medicine wheel is a Native American teaching tool. Recently it has been adapted to something called "the mistake wheel," which offers a perspective on acceptance that I find profound in experiencing happiness. The message in the north is, "Learning from our own mistakes"; the west is "Learning from the mistakes of others"; the east is "Learning from the mistakes of our teachers"; and the south is, "Being willing to make as many mistakes as it takes." Finally, in the center, which represents the pivotal learning, is "Learning that there is no such thing as a mistake."

When we see every mistake—our own or others'—as an occasion for learning, we up our happiness quotient. Yesterday I found an editing mistake I made in a book we published. My first reaction was to beat myself up. But then I stopped and asked, "What can I learn from this?" That I need more time per book, and that the world won't come to an end if I make mistakes. And if I think about in that way it is not a mistake, it is a wake-up call to realign myself with my deepest values and to devote myself only to that which I believe in passionately.

Chances are you or someone you know will make a mistake today. In what way is it not a mistake?

Try Kava Kava

Nothing makes me more cranky or lethargic than not getting my full complement of sleep the night before. For the past six years, I've had trouble sleeping, and I know firsthand it's a real happiness killer. I'm not alone—experts say one in four people have trouble sleeping, at least occasionally, and the National Commission on Sleep Disorders estimates that folks spend $16 billion a year trying to sleep. Kava kava to the rescue. Studies have shown that this South Pacific herb is as effective as Valium or Halcyon, without their side effects. A nightly dose of 150 mg not only cures insomnia in 50 percent of those trying it in as little as seven days, but it also abolishes nervousness and anxiety. Don't exceed the recommended dosage, and stay away from this supplement if you are pregnant, breastfeeding, have Parkinson's disease, are taking sedatives such as Valium (it enhances the effect; ditto for alcohol), or are allergic to pepper (it is derived from a pepper tree). Medical advice suggests you shouldn't take it for more than eight weeks at a time.

Challenge Yourself

Sometimes we are unhappy because we're stuck in a rut, bored with ourselves and our lives. That's when we need a new challenge. A challenge that is neither too easy nor too hard can really be invigorating.

A woman I work with, Suzanne, took on such a challenge to wake up her life. She decided to join the AIDS charity bike ride from San Francisco to Los Angeles, a journey of seven days and 560 miles. She rode her bike daily, and did long training rides on weekends. "I had to raise money too," she said, "$2,500, and that was the hardest part. I knew I could physically do it, but asking for money was difficult. In the end, though, I raised $5,300! That was at least as good as doing the ride itself."

You don't need to bike 560 miles or raise $5,300 to challenge yourself. What could you do that would give you a similar sense of stretching yourself? Read that long novel you've always wanted to? Take an art class? Start to work out? Give yourself a goal, and commit to it.

Take a Good Belly Breath

When we are nervous, upset, or anxious, we breathe only with the top of our chest. Some of us—myself included—actually stop breathing altogether without noticing it. Experts inform us that this shallow breathing starts around fifth grade. Before that, kids breathe calmly and deeply. No one knows quite why the change happens, but I would guess it has something to do with the onset of puberty!

Belly breathing has been shown to reduce stress and anxiety symptoms by 63 percent. Take a long slow breath in through your nose, inhaling all the way into your abdomen. Feel it rise. Then slowly let your breath out all the way, imagining the tension leaving as the air does. As you exhale, let go of the tension in your face, neck, and upper body. Relax your forehead, eyes, jaw, and tongue. Be sure to breathe slowly through the nose; breathing through your mouth can cause hyperventilation and panic attacks.

Now all you have to do is to remember to do it. Try putting a colored dot on your hand for the day. Every time you look down and see it, take a belly breath. You can do this anywhere—even in the heat of a tension-filled meeting!

What Door Is Opening?

Helen Keller once said, "When one door of happiness closes, another opens; but often we look so long at the closed door that we do not see the one which has been opened before us."

How is this true for you? Have you been hung up recently on something you've lost? What door has opened to you at the same time?

Indulge in the Arts

According to *Psychology Today*, a study of 13,000 people demonstrates that those who participate in cultural activities were less likely to die during the nine-year study than those who did not. They didn't even have to do something active—reading, or going to concerts, museums, movies and the theater all counted as much as playing a musical instrument. Researchers had many theories as to why, including that a stimulating environment may stimulate the immune system and increase brain function that may protect against depression.

What cultural or artistic endeavor calls to you? Attending a new photo exhibit? Finally learning the guitar? Swing dancing? Go for it.

Indulge in the Creature Comforts

Why do we deny ourselves so many of the creature comforts? I never buy the peach tea I love because it costs slightly more than regular tea. I can afford it, but I feel guilty indulging myself. How silly—my happiness is worth $1 a week more!

Wear that special pair of earrings, your favorite shirt, the perfume you save for special occasions. Today's special occasion is your own happiness.

How Are You Feeling?

According to Harvard University Professor Arthur Barsky, in national surveys, 46 percent of respondents say that "good health" is the greatest source of happiness, scoring higher than "great wealth" and "personal satisfaction from accomplishments." The conclusion, of course, is that if we want to be happy, we must try and stay healthy. But even if you are not completely well, an upbeat attitude can make all the difference—studies have demonstrated that people who accept their physical disabilities are far more happy than those who surrender to self-pity.

Take a moment to reflect on the good health that you do enjoy, no matter what amount that is. Can you walk with ease? See the beauty around you? Hear the sounds of the birds? Breathe freely? My father, who suffered from emphysema the last ten years of his life, always felt joyful on the days he could breath more easily. Focus on what's right about your health, and you'll feel better.

Make a Memory Box

OK, this takes a little work. But only a little. Find or buy a box you like and put your favorite things in it. Things that make you happy to hold because they bring back good memories—the picture of your newborn (he's now twenty-seven), the one earring of the pair your husband brought you from a business trip as a surprise present, the flowers from the day he told you he loved you. As the memories flood back, you will instantly feel happy.

Pay Up or Give Up

In his wonderful book *Happiness Is a Serious Matter,* Dennis Prager makes a point that I find profound. One of the secrets to happiness, he claims, is recognizing that everything has a price. And you must determine if you are willing to pay the price or let it go. A relationship has a price. So does not being in a relationship.

I know a woman who's miserable right now because she doesn't get this. She's an older woman who decided that she should go into a retirement home that guaranteed to take care of her no matter how debilitated she became. But she's depressed now because she doesn't like the location. She's not willing to pay the price of security, which in this case means living in a big-city highrise. To be happy, she must either admit to herself that she would rather have a beautiful location than lifelong security (and happily move), or acknowledge that the price of the security is worth it (and happily stay). Otherwise, she will continue to be miserable no matter what.

Is there a place in your life where you're bemoaning the price you've had to pay? As Prager says, either pay up or give it up.

Try this Irish Proverb

Count your joys instead of your woes
Count your friends instead of your foes.

That's right—count them. What are your joys? Mine in this moment are being with my daughter, swimming, reading novels, eating steak salad. So simple, really.

And friends—who are they? What do they give you? Mine offer understanding, a swift kick when necessary, laughter, and insight.

Take a News Break

We don't want to close our hearts and minds to the troubles of the world, for they affect us all, no matter where we live. But the news can be emotionally overwhelming, particularly when the news is so filled with bad things that we can begin to think that is all there is to life. A study in the British *Journal of Psychology* found that people's anxiety levels rise, even about their own personal problems, after watching negative TV news reports. That's why it is important, to keep our spirits up, to proclaim a moratorium on the news from time to time. Not to ignore what is happening, but to keep our focus on what we can do to improve ourselves, our communities, and the larger world. When we feel anxious and depressed, we lose the energy necessary to be part of the solution.

Inhale Energy

Need to put more pep into your step? Certain essential oils when inhaled activate the limbic area of your brain to stimulate your metabolism and wake up mind and body. Here's the list; try one that appeals to you: basil, cinnamon, clove, cypress, geranium, hyssop, frankincense, jasmine, marjoram, nutmeg, orange, pine, rose, sage, sandalwood, vanilla. Try a few drops on a pulse point when you feel yourself flagging.

Feed Your Mind

H. G. Wells wrote of the Buddha before he left his life of luxury to seek enlightenment that his "was the unhappiness of a fine mind that needs employment." In a word, he was bored. And boredom is a real happiness killer, for a great deal of happiness comes from the challenge of learning something new, of feeling our minds stretch around a new idea, a different perspective.

Is your mind stagnating? When was the last time you learned something that excited you? For me, I felt the flame of intellectual passion burn for the first time in a long while when I read *Navigating the Future,* which offers the skills the authors believe we will need to move through the beginning of the twenty-first century. A book, a class, a tape—stretch that mind and feel better! And remember— it's good for the body as well. Lifelong learners live 2.4 years longer than nonlearners, according to the book *Real Age.*

Look at Something Beautiful

I love to look at my daughter and my husband. Both of them, in my eyes, are beautiful, and I never fail to get an emotional rush when I gaze at either of them. What gives you that special lift? A loved one, a pet? The photograph in your bedroom? The needlepoint pillow your mother gave you? Today, look around your home and feast your eyes on one thing that gives you joy.

What Do You Really Need?

Needs and wants are different. Wants left unchecked lead to dissatisfaction because there are always more than can be satisfied. We can't have all our desires—if only because the strain on the Earth is too much. If we let our desires run wild, we will be disappointed and unhappy. One thing I do when I find myself running amok wanting things is to ask myself, "Do I really need this to be happy?" Most often the answer is no.

But we do have legitimate needs that must be fulfilled for us to be happy. The needs may be different for each of us, but it's important that we know what they are, so that we don't get so caught up in feeding our desires and neglect our true needs.

What do you really need to be happy? Right now, this is my list: Loving relationships, work with meaning. What about you?

What Do You Need Right Now?

At any given moment, on any given day, we need certain things and not others. What is true for you today? Do you crave excitement? Sleep? More intellectual stimulation? Ask yourself the question, "What do I need right now?" and see what the answer is. Can you give yourself a bit of it, even for a few minutes today?

Value Growth

One of the happiest people I know is my friend Dawna. She's had many health difficulties in her life, which only makes her sunny attitude that much more remarkable. I've studied her for ten years now, and I finally realized that she is happy because she values growth. She sees life as a giant experiment in learning, and no matter what befalls her, she asks herself what kind of growth is being called for.

When we value emotional and spiritual growth, life's ups and downs have meaning; instead of bemoaning our fate, we can use every opportunity to become more of who we are meant to be. For you, that might mean becoming more assertive; for me, trusting more. But for both of us, whatever hardship we're facing can become an occasion for growth.

Where are you being called on to stretch beyond your current limits? Can you see the challenge as a chance for growth?

Indulge in Dinner

It's easy to get the winter blues. When I lived in Ithaca, New York, it could be overcast for six weeks at a time or longer during the winter. By February I was nearly suicidal.

To combat the winter blues, take the opportunity tonight to indulge yourself with a really good dinner. Make your favorite food. Buy fresh flowers, use cloth napkins, light a scented candle. Go all out for no reason except uplifting your spirits.

Lose Yourself

I recently came across an article in *New Age* magazine by Bob Genovesi in which he was counseling a depressed friend to find something to be passionate about. He said, "To be happy with yourself, you've got to lose yourself now and then."

I couldn't agree more! We can get so obsessed with ourselves, with our pain, with how others have slighted us, how life is screwing us over. Sometimes we need to quit wallowing and get involved with something that lets us forget ourselves for a while. It could be anything—painting, model airplane building, teaching reading to illiterate adults—all that is required is that you care enough about it to let yourself be absorbed for awhile.

When I was in the midst of a painful breakup, my friend Daphne counseled me to go out and volunteer. Once a week for two years I delivered meals to people with AIDS and always found it to be emotionally uplifting. How can you lose yourself?

Do Something You Love Today—
Even Only for Five Minutes

What gives you great pleasure that you haven't experienced in a while? Going to the movies and eating a large bucket of popcorn? Reading a trashy book? Calling a long-distance friend? Making love? Whatever it is, give yourself permission to indulge today.

Notice What's Right

We can make ourselves miserable or happy in any given moment by choosing to focus on what's wrong, or choosing to focus on what's right. There is always plenty of both. We can notice what's missing, what's broken, what's imperfect—and make ourselves miserable. Try it right now. Make a mental list of all the ways your life is imperfect: Your spouse forgets your anniversary, your child is not an A student; your boss is less than complimentary. Life sucks!

Now, turn it around and focus on what's right, with the exact same people: Your spouse greets you at the end of every day with a big hug and kiss; your child is great at making friends; your boss gives you a great deal of autonomy, proving she trusts you. Life is pretty good!

In any given situation, you can shine the light on what's right or what's wrong. For today, notice what's working and see how you feel.

Buy a Wind Chime

According to music researcher Stephen Halpern, Ph.D., certain wind chimes produce harmonious, soothing sounds that can actually lower your breathing and heart rate, increasing calm and contentment. Test it out: Strike a chime a few times and notice if your breath slows as you listen.

Drop the Blame Game

I learned this lesson early on in my work life from my partner Will Glennon, and it has been a great skill for harmony and happiness. When a mistake is made, fix it as best you can and move on. Getting caught in the "It's your fault; no it isn't, I'm blameless" game is a terrible energy drain. Better to use that same energy to find a solution. Sometimes the solution lies in fixing the immediate error; other times it lies in creating a new system to prevent the mistake from happening again; and sometimes both approaches are required. Nothing is served by spending a lot of time hand-wringing and finger-pointing except anger and guilt.

Are you caught in the blame game somewhere in your life? At home with your spouse? At work? When things are tough, finger-pointing is very tempting. But resist the temptation, and your life will be infinitely happier. If you find it hard to let go, say to yourself, "We're all doing the best we can."

Do a Shoulder Shrug

The tension we hold in our bodies is a big happiness vacuum. While it is possible to be happy and in pain, it certainly isn't desirable. Most of the time we override our body's signals, ignoring its cries for attention and relief.

I suggest that at least three times today you do shoulder shrugs, preferably when you notice the tension building in your upper back as you work. It's incredibly easy—and feels great. With your hands in your lap or by your sides, simply lift your shoulders toward your ears as high as they will go, hold for five seconds, then let your shoulders drop, exhaling audibly. (You can skip the noise if you are in a meeting.) Repeat five times. Doesn't that feel great?

Commit to Loving Better

Today, in honor of the day devoted to love, take the love pledge: "I open to more love today, more love of myself and those I meet in my day. I commit to giving without worry about receiving." Then notice what changes in your life as a consequence.

Have a Brazil Nut

One Brazil nut contains the recommended daily allowance of selenium, a mineral that has been found to boost spirits. It can also be found in chicken, seafood, and whole grains. If you want to be sure you're getting enough, consider a supplement; 55 mg per day should do it.

Sleep Well

If you, like me, spend many a night tossing and turning, you might want to consider your diet as the culprit. Here's how: carbohydrates send tryptophan, an amino acid known to be a sleep aid, to the brain, while protein actually inhibits trytophan's sedative effect. So avoid high-protein dinners and try carbo loading before bedtime. Or you may be mineral deficient; iron, calcium and magnesium all induce sleepiness. Try taking those supplements in the evening. Hunger can also keep you awake—maybe you're not eating enough (but don't overdo either; overeating can cause stomach pains that will keep you awake). And finally, maybe you're drinking too much alcohol. A drink can help you go to sleep, but it often causes wakefulness in the middle of the night and can interfere with the body's REM cycle, which is when the most restful sleep occurs.

Greet the Day

How we begin the morning sets the tone for the whole day. If we drag out of bed grumbling, chances are we will have trouble feeling happy during the day. In many cultures, greeting the sun is part of spiritual practice, a way of beginning in gratitude and awe for the new day we've been given. In her wise and warm book *The Woman's Book of Spirit,* Sue Patton Thoele has a wonderful meditation for greeting the new day that is sure to get your morning off to the right start:

"Close your eyes and imagine yourself waking. How do you normally feel? Are you happy with the way you greet the day? If the answer is no, imagine how you would like to change your greeting. Are you smiling? What do you say? Slowly, gently visualize yourself, in the perfect right time and way, awaken to the gift of a pure, new day. Greet it in the fresh way that you imagined. How does that feel?"

Try DLPA

DLPA is a natural supplement recommended by Dr. Andrew Weil and other natural health experts as a pain-killer and depression lifter. Researchers claim that 24 million women battle depression every year, and that 74 percent could get relief in as short a time as a week by taking 200 mg of DLPA per day. DLPA is a combination of amino acids found in peas, lentils, and other protein-rich foods that is known to elevate blood levels of norepinephrine and the body's other natural mood elevators. It's available at nutrition and health food stores and should be taken half before breakfast and half before lunch. "For best absorption," says Dr. Weil, "take it with 500 mg of vitamin C, 100 mg of vitamin B6, and a glass of juice." It is not recommended for pregnant and breastfeeding women. Check with your doctor if you have high blood pressure or other medical disorders. Non-habit-forming, the only known side effect is slight jitters in some people.

Acknowledge the Truth
of the Moment

I've come to believe that much of our misery comes from not being willing to acknowledge the truth of the present circumstance. We wish it weren't so; we want things to be different, so we either deny what is really going on or complain that it shouldn't be the way it is.

I've found so much peace of mind from just acknowledging the plain truth, whatever it is, no matter how hard: right now, our relationship is going through a rough patch; right now, the stepkids are having a hard time adjusting to the new baby their father and I had; in this moment I feel totally lost. Depending on the circumstance, sometimes I just say it to myself; other times I share it with the other person involved. The truth of this moment is just that: the truth of this moment. It says nothing about the next moment, the next day, or the next year. And as the old adage says, the truth will set you free.

That's because it encourages us to get out of denial or grousing and acknowledge what is true for us right now. By naming it, we can begin to tame it, as my friend Dawna says. If only by recognizing that what is true now may not be true later.

What is your truth of the moment?

Fix What's Bugging You

In *Learned Optimism,* Martin Seligman offers research to show that the main difference between happy, successful people and depressed, unsuccessful folks is how they deal with difficulty. Unhappy people tend to shut down in the face of a problem; happy individuals take action to solve their problems. Optimists also tend not to get mired in blaming themselves for what's wrong as pessimists do; they focus instead on solutions.

If, like me, you're not a natural optimist, you still can cultivate the mental attitudes of one—or at least tone down your negative thinking. When you find yourself getting mired in a problem, say to yourself, "I can fix this." Rather than complaining, make a list of ten things (no matter how crazy) you can do to help solve the situation. For example, if you are concerned about money, here's a list of things you can do to generate more: rent a room in your house, baby-sit at night, sell your used books, sell your car, start day trading, have your child become a model, offer to barter instead of paying cash for things, pay your mortgage bimonthly (it's shaving three years off my thirty-year mortgage—a huge savings), go to night school and learn a trade, grow plants and vegetables and sell them at the farmer's market. Then look at the list and see what makes the most sense. Try it.

Give a Compliment Today

I was reminded about the importance of compliments recently when my coworker and I were having a typically stressful day and handling twenty-five things at once, strategizing how to handle the various upsets swirling around us, when it suddenly popped into my mind to say how much I enjoyed working with her. Her smile went from ear to ear, and so did mine.

Saying something nice to someone is not only a great spirit lifter for the other person, but for you as well. There is nothing like the high that comes from brightening someone else's day.

Compliments have an great side effect too. The more you say wonderful things about people, the more you are perceived of as being wonderful. The converse is also true—the more you gossip, say, about someone's infidelity, the more you yourself are perceived as a philanderer. It's not logical, but studies have shown that gossips are seen as having the same qualities as those they are gossiping about.

Make someone's day—and yours—by giving them a compliment.

Focus on Your Own Success

Recently an acquaintance of mine got a book advance of half a million dollars. That is a lot of money. I found myself green with envy, and full of negative self-talk—What am I doing wrong? Why can't I ever get a break? I spiraled right down into a black hole.

Then I remembered that life is not a contest with one grand prize winner at the end. Simply because another person has succeeded doesn't mean you've failed. In fact, it says nothing about your success or failure at all.

The incident made me reflect on what success really means to me. How do I measure success? By money? Does the person with the most toys win? I know in my heart that is shallow. By fame? I don't truly care about being famous. I realized that I would consider myself successful in my own life if I loved well and made a difference in the world through my books. On both those scores, I can consider myself successful.

What is true success to you?

Envision What You Want

This morning, before you start your day, use the power of visualization to create a day full of joy. See yourself handling the difficulties of your work life with equanimity. See yourself smiling at each person you meet, treating each person with care and kindness. See yourself as the calm in the center of the storm of life. Then notice how the day goes. Are you happier as a consequence?

Let Your Mind Wander

Most of us spend so many of our working hours on focused mental activities—thinking about specific problems and solutions. Our minds never get a vacation except when they are asleep. But our minds need time off too. We need to be able to "space out" every day, to get wide and wondering, rather than just concentrated and alert. Because that's where new ideas are generated, where we find the creative solutions to the problems plaguing us, where we reconnect to what is most deeply important to our souls.

For just five minutes today, indulge in the pleasure of mental meandering. I like to do it when I'm driving. I just let my mind go wherever it wants, with no goal in mind. Sometimes I'm not even aware of thinking at all. Some part of my mind is driving carefully; the rest is who knows where. I get my best ideas that way.

Make a Play Date

My friend Daphne and I love to play dress up. We go shopping for fun and often don't buy a thing. We just spend a few hours putting on clothes and seeing how we look in them. Ball gowns are particularly enjoyable; just the other day we found the perfect thing for her to wear to the Academy Awards, if she were ever invited. She looked just like Marilyn Monroe at JFK's birthday party.

How do you like to play? Mountain biking? Wind surfing? Going to a spa and having a facial? Do something that you consider play today.

Seek Out a Third Place

Sometimes all we need is a change of environment to lift our spirits. We can get so stuck in traversing the path from home to work and back that we don't venture any further. But for years, scientists have touted the benefits of what sociologist Georg Simmel calls your "third place"—a public venue where you can "stand outside yourself and get some perspective." Some people find their third place in cafés, others in public parks. Some folks like the anonymous buzz of people around them; others need solitude. (An author I know once did a research project in which she asked students to name the places in nature they went to for comfort. As I remember, they fell into two categories—those near water, and those that afforded a long view. A young man in the Midwest, which is very flat, chose the top of a tower.)

Do you have a third place? If so, make some time for it soon. If not, imagine the benefits of finding one.

Be the Sky

This is a practice that was very useful to me when I was going through hard times and feeling overwhelmed by sadness and loss. It comes from the Vietnamese Buddhist monk Thich Nhat Hanh, one of the wisest and happiest beings I've ever encountered.

Whenever I'm feeling badly, for any reason, I sit quietly for a few minutes and imagine myself as the wide blue sky and my feelings as clouds moving across the sky. In doing so, I remind myself that I, myself, am bigger than the feelings. That the feelings are moving through me rather than taking me over. That my essence is vast, unchanging, eternal, while the feelings are temporary and transitory. No matter what is going on, I always feel more peaceful afterward.

See if it works for you.

Take Charge with a Small Action

If home or work life seems overwhelming, it's easy to sink into depression or despair. It all feels like too much, so you do nothing.

The truth is you can turn your mood around by taking charge with a small action. Turn the ringer off the phone, clear out all your e-mail, make that one call you've been dreading. When you take control of the situation by managing even a little bit of your environment you feel better. For example, in a study done by psychologist Judith Rodin, 93 percent of residents at a nursing home got happier when they were allowed to make policy decisions at the home. That helped them feel more in control and therefore happier.

Where can you take charge right now?

Picture Yourself Happier

Jody Friedman is a New York psychoanalyst who does photoanalysis with her clients by having them bring in pictures of themselves as youngsters to help them tap into their deepest desires. Here's how to do it on your own:

1. Choose a full-body photo of yourself between the ages of two and twelve that you like;

2. Imagine what the child in that photo would do if no one was there to say no;

3. Whatever the answer is, ask yourself, "How can I bring more of that into my life?"

4. Visualize yourself doing it.

Talk Nicely to Your Significant Other for One Minute

Want a happy relationship? Couples therapist John Gottman discovered that one minute of expressing appreciation for the other person before launching into a difficult topic made the difference between whether people felt happy in their relationships or ended up getting divorced. The happiest couples expressed positive feelings thirty seconds longer than those who felt they had a moderately happy marriage, and moderately happy couples were positive thirty seconds longer than those who later divorced. So take a minute to appreciate your loved one—aren't they worth it?

Find a Slogan

Whenever I am going through a hard place, I like to tape an inspiring quote on my computer to cheer me up or remind me of something I tend to forget when in the doldrums. For months, when I was feeling stuck at work, I used a Henry Miller quote: "Life is constantly providing us with new funds, new resources, even when we are reduced to immobility. In life's ledger there is no such thing as frozen assets." I would be sitting there feeling stuck, look at Miller's words, and find my spirit lifting as I imagined life working behind the scenes on my behalf, making things happen to change the circumstances.

These days, my slogan is from Dawna Markova: "Wherever you are is meaningful and the beginning of something else." Just typing it now cheers me up.

Try it—but it has to be something that has meaning for you. There are a gazillion quotation books, or check out some quote sites on the Internet. The one I use is **quips-subscribe@topica.com**.

Climb Out of the Money Pit

Money brings some happiness. But after a certain point,
it just brings more money.
—Neil Simon

It's so easy to get fooled into thinking that money will buy happiness. In a *New York Times* article dated February 2, 1999, the reporter reviewed recent psychological studies that substantiate the adage that money can't buy happiness: "Not only does having more things prove to be unfulfilling, but people for whom affluence is a priority in life tend to experience an unusual degree of anxiety and depression as well as a lower overall level of well-being."

To get out of the money pit, try this meditation adapted from *Living a Sacred Life* by Robin Heerens Lysne: Sit in a comfortable chair. Affirm, "I am taken care of by God (or my Higher Power, the Universe, or whatever feels right to you). I am nurtured and loved and all my basic needs are met."

B Well!

Researchers have found a connection between depression and B-vitamin deficiencies, and many of us, particularly those who are watching their weight, don't get enough Bs. To compensate, try a B-complex vitamin pill, or load up on kidney, lima, and garbanzo beans. Beans are a great source of B vitamins (and they are good in the fiber department too!).

If you are looking for a way to take vitamins without breaking your bank account, look at **www.healthshop.com, www.mothernature.com,** and **www.vitaminshoppe.com**. They all offer vitamins, minerals, herbs, and other supplements at deep discounts.

Turn on Soothing Sounds

Some noises are actually good for you. The tinkling of water in a fountain, and the white noise of a humidifier or fan have been found to lower your heart rate and raise the endorphin levels that make you feel good.

I discovered this trick years ago. As a teen, I used to have trouble falling asleep. But one summer, I realized that sleep came easily when the fan was on in my room to try to relieve the August heat. It worked so well that I used it for months afterward, pointing the fan away from my bed. Then one day in November, my father heard the noise and came in and took it away. Many years later, I rediscovered this magic when we installed a humidifier in our bedroom. I've been sleeping—and dreaming—much more soundly.

You don't need to wait for nightfall—a table fountain is a wonderful stress buster you can enjoy throughout your day.

Find Your Purpose

This is the true joy of life, being used up for a purpose recognized by yourself as a mighty one; being a force of nature instead of a feverish, selfish little clot of ailments and grievances, complaining that the world will not devote itself to making you happy.

—George Bernard Shaw

In *Flow,* University of California professor Mihily Csikszentmihalyi describes research that he and colleagues have done on happiness. Subjects carried beepers and were beeped about eight times a day. When they were beeped, they were to write down what they were doing and how they felt. The researchers discovered that people were most happy while engaged in something meaningful to them.

Nothing is more meaningful than feeling you are being used for a deep purpose. But I know many people who have a hard time figuring out what their purpose is. If you too are wondering, ask yourself the two great questions: "What am I here to give? What am I here to learn?" Your purpose can be found in your answers.

Cultivate Situational Optimism

For the past couple of decades, researchers and writers such as Norman Cousins and Bernie Siegel have touted the health and happiness benefits of a positive attitude. But you are either an optimist or a pessimist and can't do a whole lot to change that, right? Wrong. Recently, scientists have begun to differentiate between dispositional optimists (those who look on the bright side in general) and situational optimists (those who use positive thinking for an immediate challenge). What they found is that though both types of optimism strengthen the immune system, the biggest rise in T-cell and killer cell levels (measures of the strength of the immune system) was seen in situational optimists. And the even better news is that situational optimism can be learned. (I am living proof!)

What doesn't work is to tell a natural pessimist to look on the bright side. What is effective is to tell yourself, when faced with a challenge, "I have the capacity to deal effectively with this. What positive step can I take right now to reach a good outcome?"

Take Time Alone Today

All human evil comes from this:
a person's being unable to sit still in a room.

—Pascal

MARCH
9

Solitude is good for you—at least occasionally. Psychologists have discovered that while long periods of isolation can be unhealthy, one hour alone in a darkened flotation tank results in greater creativity, lower blood pressure, improved mental function, and a more positive outlook on life.

Can you steal some alone time today?

Coaxing Spring

Right about now, chances are you've got the winter blahs. For an easy pick-me-up, anticipate spring by forcing flower branches to bring a bit of color indoors. Any of a wide variety of bushes, shrubs, and trees will do, including forsythia, crab apple, pussy willow, quince, plum, cherry, dogwood, privet, red maple, gooseberry, weeping willow, or witch hazel. Simply cut the edges of the branches on a slant with sharp scissors and plunge immediately into a vase of warm water. Change the water every few days, and the warmth of the house will do the rest of the work. Instant spring!

The Loving Kindness Meditation

I consider myself a Buddhist, but I am a terrible meditator. I can't seem to find the time to sit for even ten minutes a day. But I do have a daily practice that brings me incredible tranquility and joy. Nowadays I do it with my two-year-old as I put her to sleep. It's called "Loving Kindness Meditation," and it's about wishing well to yourself, those you know and love, and all beings.

There are many different formulas, but here's what I do: Sit or lie down quietly and say aloud or to yourself, "May I be peaceful. May I be happy. May I be free from suffering. May I be filled with loving kindness." Then bring someone close to you to mind and say the same to him or her: "May Ana be peaceful. May she be happy. May she be free from suffering. May she be filled with loving kindness." Keep on going until you have included everyone you want to, moving from those close to you and ending with everyone: "May all beings be peaceful. May all beings be happy. May all beings be free from suffering."

I like to do it when I am upset with someone (it often transforms the feelings immediately because it puts me in touch with my caring for them), or when I'm feeling powerless (for example, to prevent war or starvation). This offering of good wishes has done more than anything else to increase my happiness.

Remember We Are Love in Motion

*We forget that if we don't show up, somebody, even one
somebody, would miss what we had to offer, ask, or do
that day. We do not recognize that we are love in motion,
seeking to reveal itself in many ways under all circumstances.*

—Iyanla Vanzant

As Iyanla Vanzant reminds us, we can get so fixated on
what's wrong in our lives or what we have to do to keep the
daily round going that we forget that we are all here to
love. We lose sight of the fact that just the mere fact of our
being in the world, no matter what our circumstances, can
and does matter. Because we were standing there, our child
didn't get hit by a car. Because we showed up at work, a
new idea was generated that might help countless people.
Because we listened, our mother's heart was soothed, if
only for a few hours. Every day offers us countless opportunities to love— the homeless man in the street, the
woman behind the deli counter, the friends and loved ones
that grace our lives.

What would happen if you thought of yourself as love
in motion today?

Watch an Uplifting Movie

In *The Little Book of Big Questions,* Jonathan Robinson polled hundreds of people as to what movies they found most inspiring. From that list and my informal poll, here's the top twenty in alphabetical order: *Babette's Feast; Being There; Brother Sun, Sister Moon; Chariots of Fire; Dances with Wolves; Dead Poets Society; Forrest Gump; Gandhi; Grand Canyon; Groundhog Day; Harold and Maude; Hearts and Souls; Like Water for Chocolate; E.T.; Life Is Beautiful; Out of Africa; Philadelphia; The Razor's Edge; Resurrection; Schindler's List.* Rent one tonight, and don't forget the popcorn.

Take a Peace Break

Rather than refueling with caffeine, which can cause jitters and insomnia, why not take periodic "peace" breaks to consciously breathe and come back to yourself? You can do it in the bathroom, or using the phone as a trigger— every time it rings, use the bell as a reminder to breathe, and then pick up the receiver on the third ring. Or you can even use the computer as your helper. Log on to a cyper-meditation room where you can watch fluffy clouds float by as you breathe. Try **www.calmcentre.com/meditation room.html**.

Put the Pressure On—Your Feet

Reflexology is a method of applying pressure to certain points on your foot to relieve stress and promote health. The theory is that different places on the foot correspond to various organs and bodily systems. The massage described below works the endocrine system, which is responsible for, among other things, our moods and mental well-being. This is a great stress reliever and mood elevator.

Hold your right foot with your left hand. Press with your right thumb up the big toe as shown below. Repeat three times. Switch feet.

And if you don't want to go through the trouble of doing it yourself, consider Rockport Shoes' new line of shoes based on reflexology—they are equipped with air pockets to massage certain points as you walk.

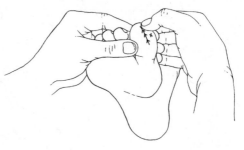

Reel in Road Rage

Road rage has become an increasing problem as we spend more and more of our scarce time driving on overcrowded highways. Since most of us have to drive a lot (commutes are now an hour on average), we might as well learn the skills to drive happily in any situation. Here are three suggestions from Leon James, Ph.D., creator of the video course *RoadRageous:*

Defuse your anger by counting slowly or singing.

Create as pleasant an experience as possible—listen to a book on tape or your favorite music; buy a pair of beautiful driving gloves or padded seat.

Don't assume that other drivers' mistakes are intentional.

Other ideas: tell yourself you have enough time to get where you are going, no matter how long it takes; practice a random act of kindness by letting other cars cut in or pass if they want to; leave earlier so that you don't freak out if there is a traffic snag.

Try aromatherapy. Aveda (**www.aveda.com**) now has calming car scents in a kit called Air & Body Care Airmobile Kit.

Ask Yourself, "So What?"

In his children's book, *The Meanest Thing to Say,* comic
Bill Cosby reveals the best retort to any insult: "So?" It's
good advice for adults as well.

Today, when you find yourself stressing over something, ask yourself, "So what?" So what if the report is late?
So what if I don't answer every e-mail? So what if I leave
something until tomorrow? "So what?" gets you back on
track to focus on what's most important to you.

Serve Yourself Well

Have you ever had truly gracious service from a waiter? A customer service person? What if you treated yourself just as well right now? What if you gently inquired if there was anything you needed and then quickly went off to get whatever was required?

As Sue Patton Thoele says in *The Woman's Book of Confidence,* "For this one day—which, hopefully, will stretch into a lifetime—make it your joy and privilege to ask yourself, 'What can I get you to make this day better? How may I serve you right now?'"

We all deserve to be treated well, especially by ourselves.

Will This Make Me Happy?

Just for today, before making any decision, big or small, ask yourself, "Will this make me happy?" Will buying this sweater, calling this person, having this meeting, make me happy? If the answer is yes, do it. If not, don't. At the end of the day, notice how you feel and how your day was different.

Surround Yourself with Good Smells

I've always been a bit doubtful about aromatherapy. I knew that certain smells made me feel good emotionally, but how could certain smells be good for me physically? I guess I was forgetting the old mind-body connection. Recent research in England actually shows a correlation between smells and the effectiveness of the immune system as measured by a certain antibody in the bloodstream. A bad smell (rotten meat) caused the antibody level to be suppressed, while a good smell (chocolate) caused it to increase.

So today, indulge yourself in a favorite scent. For me, it's Shalimar. For my husband, tuberoses. Not only will you feel happier, your body will feel better too.

Count Your Thoughts

This one takes a bit of practice, but you can get the benefit from it even if you succeed just a little bit. Because happiness is an inside job, and because it has been shown that we are constantly sending either positive or negative messages to ourselves, people who are happy have predominately positive thoughts. Therefore, to be happier, we need to learn to increase the number of positive thoughts and decrease the negative ones.

For today, count the number of negative and positive thoughts you have in ten minutes. The trick is to notice yourself thinking; so much of this is below the level of consciousness. But the more you intend to notice, the more you will notice. It's easiest to do when nothing else is going on. So sit down quietly and notice where you mind goes. Does it beat you up for forgetting to notice your thinking? Does it habitually go toward gloomy possibilities?

Doing this was very powerful for me. I realized that in ten minutes, I had only negative thoughts—castigating myself, worrying about the future turning out badly. I did not think one positive thing! If your mind is deeply grooved in negativity, it won't go away overnight. What I've learned to do is that when I notice myself looking on the dark side, I consciously think a few positive thoughts as well to counteract it.

That May Not Be True

Yesterday we looked at the kind of negative self-talk we engage in on a regular basis. Today we're going to explore further how to counteract it. The good news is that you can learn to be more positive and optimistic. In studies, children who were put through the Penn Optimism Program were less likely to be depressed, and those with depressive symptoms cut their risk in half.

What did they do? First they learned to identify their negative thinking, and then they learned to say to themselves, "Wait a minute! That may not be true." Here's an example: A child gets a D on a test. The negative thought is "I'm stupid." The child is taught to think of alternate explanations and reframings: "I did well last time. Just because I did poorly on one test doesn't mean I'm stupid." Give it a try. When you catch yourself making a negative statement about yourself or someone else, think of alternate positive explanations.

Plant Good Wishes

In *Living a Sacred Life,* author Robin Heerens Lysne has a great suggestion for a springtime ritual that you can do with young children. Take some paperwhite narcissus, daffodils, or other spring bulbs and plant them in a bowl full of pebbles. As you place each bulb, make a wish for the spring. Fill bowl with water, and watch over the weeks as your wishes blossom.

Take a Satisfaction Break

We can get so caught up in the rat race of our lives that we never take the time to appreciate our accomplishments. That was certainly true for me, even as a child—I got an A on the test, but I was always focused on the next test or the next course. When I had a bestselling book, I was busy focusing on the next book: Would it do as well? As a consequence, I never got to experience the happiness that comes from meeting a goal. I just raced onto the next one. One day, my friend Dawna said to me, "You need to take a satisfaction break. Yes, you have more to do. But right now, can't you enjoy what you have already done?" Her words rang in my ears.

So how about taking a satisfaction break right now? Make a list of the accomplishments you are proudest of, and then read over your list and appreciate yourself for all your hard work. You've done a lot, so celebrate already!

Wave at a Child

H. Jackson Brown, Jr., the bestselling author of *Life's Little Instruction Book,* is great at reminding us of the simple things that can bring joy and happiness. I've adapted one of his ideas:

Today, while driving, wave to the kids you come across. If you see a schoolbus or van, great. Otherwise, wave to the kids in cars going or coming from school. You'll feel better, honest.

Acknowledge Anger

*Speak when you are angry and
you will make the best speech you will ever regret.*
—Ambrose Bierce

As researchers learn more and more about the human body, it has become clearer and clearer that both blowing up in anger and stifling it are bad for you—emotionally and physically (not to mention what it does to the other person). Recently, scientists at Ohio State University discovered that both tactics led to elevated levels of LDL, the "bad" cholesterol that damages arteries and leads to strokes and heart attacks. However, folks who were able to calmly express their feelings at the appropriate time had 10 percent lower LDLs than those who exploded or repressed.

If you can't express your feelings calmly, follow the advice of Iyanla Vanzant and KYBYS (Keep Your Big Yap Shut) until you can. Count to ten, one hundred, or one thousand. But don't express until you can do it without a double-barrel shotgun.

Check Out These Sleep Remedies

For all of these, read the labels and follow the directions. As usual, consult a doctor before taking any remedy. And don't take them all at once—it will be too hard to tell which is effective. Try one after another until you hit on what works for you.

Passion flower—tea or extract;

Valerian—tea or supplements;

The homeopathic remedy gelsemium for relieving anxiety that leads to sleeplessness.

Engage Your Empathy

I've never been a big fan of *A Course in Miracles,* but recently I came across something from it that is the wisest thing I've heard in a long time: "The worse people act, the greater is their need for healing."

I can't tell you how useful that has been for me to remember. Now, when someone is verbally attacking me or when I learn about backbiting comments someone has made, instead of shutting down, running, or attacking back, I can engage my empathy. I realize the pain they must be in to behave in such a manner, and I can offer my silent wishes that they be healed. On occasion, I've even applied it to myself. When I find myself behaving in a less than stellar way, instead of collapsing in shame, I acknowledge my need for healing and apologize.

Increasing my caring for others under stress rather than shutting them up or down allows me to stay connected to my heart and to the other person, and has defused many a volatile situation. Perhaps it will work for you too.

Watch the Sunrise or Sunset

It doesn't matter which you choose, although sometimes it's more fun to pick the one you usually don't see. But this time, really watch it. Not as the backdrop to your life, but at least for the moment, as the main event.

MARCH
29

Hold a Pity Party

I love this idea. It comes from Paul Pearsall's book *Write Your Own Pleasure Prescription.* "Healthy balance is not just being up, staying strong, and having a stiff upper lip; it also means making space for less pleasant emotions. Set a timer for ten minutes and have a short pity party for yourself. . . . Go ahead and feel very sorry for yourself. Intentionally pout your lower lip. Look sad for your full ten minutes [and indulge in all the reasons you have to feel sorry for yourself], and then put on a happier face when your timer goes off, even if you have to fake it. Just smiling will cause a little positive emotional spurt."

Be Willing to Ask for Help

None of us can make it in life, at least not happily, completely on our own. We are social creatures designed to give and receive support. In this moment, what do you need help with in order to increase your happiness? Is it housework help? Help meeting a deadline? Advice for finding a new career?

We make ourselves miserable by trying to go it all alone. And we drive ourselves and others crazy by assuming they should automatically know what we need without our having to ask for it. Ask for what you need today, and you're more likely to receive it.

Rent a Funny Video

April is National Humor Month, and today is April Fool's Day, so of course laughing is in order.

Laughing is good for you—laughing increases good hormones and decreases bad ones. You don't even have to watch a whole comedy. Researchers at Cornell University have discovered that watching even five minutes of a funny movie made people feel happier. Get a really funny video and receive the added benefit of some couch exercise—supposedly 100 belly laughs is the equivalent of exercising for ten minutes.

Exercise

Ugh! I hate exercise, and frankly I usually feel too tired to do it (I'm not alone—a study by Penn State discovered that fatigue is the reason given by 70 percent of people who fail to exercise regularly). But the truth is that exercise is just what we need to feel good—increased blood flow from exercise oxygenates the body and makes you feel more energized.

Researchers at the University of Georgia recently discovered that exercise reduces anxiety better than resting. It offers a time out from worries and gives us an energy boost that enhances a sense of well-being. Moderate activity is all that's required—walking, swimming, dancing, or gardening thirty minutes a day. Do it in ten-minute increments—a ten-minute walk to the corner, a run up three flights of stairs. If you have trouble sleeping, do some exercise at least five hours before going to bed.

I'll do it today if you will.

Embrace Enthusiasm

Young kids are full of such boundless wonder and enthusiasm. Sadly, many of us have had this natural zest for living squelched in the process of growing up. But it is possible to re-access this natural energy booster with a meditation taken from Sue Patton Thoele's *The Woman's Book of Spirit:*

"Close your eyes and allow yourself to sink deeply into the very center of your being. Focus on your breath and allow it to become slower and deeper.... Imagine ... you see a beautiful Being walking down a shaft of moonlight.... With complete candor, you begin to share with this Being your dreams, aspirations, and just-plain-fun ideas. She listens with unbounded enthusiasm.... Bask in the warmth of her attention and enthusiasm for your thoughts. Feel yourself becoming inspired and creative as a result.

"Today, if only for a few minutes, allow yourself to be possessed by this divinely enthusiastic spirit. Search out at least one thing about which you can unabashedly gush. I bet you'll be surprised how infectious your excitement is to others and how energized you feel as a result."

Get a Life

A recent study conducted at Carnegie Mellon University found that people who excel at work don't work longer than other people. What's the difference between the over-achievers and the rest of the working population? Those who excel have a life outside of work, which makes them happier, more rested, and therefore, more efficient.

Do you spend all your waking hours working? What small change could you make to bring more balance, and therefore more contentment, into your life?

Beware of Emotional Vampires

Emotional vampires are people who suck the energy out of you or otherwise bring you down. They do it in various ways—by endlessly complaining, general negativity, badmouthing others (my experience with badmouthers: you'll be the target as soon as you leave the room). We tend to take on the energy charge of those whom we are around, so the more time you spend with vampires, the more depressed and negative you'll feel.

Do yourself a favor and avoid spending a lot of time with people who bring you down. Instead, focus on folks who are like rays of sunshine in your life, and soon you'll be shining too.

Give Yourself an April Shower

From *Living a Sacred Life:* "Today, begin your shower giving thanks to the water, giving thanks to the air that you breathe, and, standing in the shower, imagine that it is blessing you. Imagine one or two things that you want to release, set your intention, and let the water carry them away. Continue the release process as you dry yourself off."

Mental Snooze Inducers

Do you find yourself unable to sleep because a hundred thoughts are crowding your brain? Or maybe you are like me—you go to sleep fine, then wake up some time in the middle of the night when your brain flashes on like a thousand-watt bulb. Here are some tricks for coping:

- Turn the clock so you can't see what time it is. Knowing only makes you more anxious.
- Read something boring—a dense history book filled with dates or a computer manual.
- Make a list of the thoughts running through your brain so you can let them go.
- Leave your thoughts by concentrating on your heartbeat and listening to every breath.

Identify Your Hot Buttons

What drives you around the bend, makes you crazy, sends you to the moon? If you take the time to make a list of your biggest bugaboos, you will be able to think about ways to eliminate or at least minimize them, rather than just complain about them.

Does clutter around the house drive you to distraction? Hold a throwaway party next Saturday, when everyone in the house goes through closets and rooms and gets rid of everything they've outgrown mentally or physically. (Donate the items to charity.) Buy or make new storage containers and make each person, child or adult, responsible for a two-minute pick-up of their stuff before going to bed.

Of maybe it's the traffic jams you seem to spend much of your life battling. Can you move closer to work? Take mass transit? Work at home a couple days a week? Get a new job? Don't just assume that no other options are possible—where there's a will there's (almost always) a way. And remember that it may involve compromises—a job with less stress and less money, for example. Focus with a constructive eye on what's making you miserable, and you'll soon be feeling much better.

Schedule a Seven-Pillow Princess (or Prince) Day

The Seven-Pillow Princess Day is one in which you stay in bed all day (if that appeals to you). It takes a bit of preparation, not only to find the time to goof off, but to stock up on the supplies you'll need: the books or magazines you've been longing to read, precisely the food you want to eat in bed, a journal to write or draw in, polish to paint your toenails, favorite videos, and plenty of bolsters and pillows in which to luxuriate.

APRIL

9

The point is to have a totally self-indulgent, lying-around kind of day in which you stay in bed as long as you want, doing exactly what you want, eating only what you want. (No diets allowed!) It's a great antidote to too much flying around and attending to other people's needs. Instead, you pretend you're a princess or prince, and cater to your every whim. If you've got kids or a spouse, schedule one for each of you on different weekends and take turns being the baby-sitter. Believe me, it will do your heart, mind, and body good!

Do the Telephone Meditation

This wonderful happiness booster for you and those you speak to comes from Thich Nhat Hanh. Today, when the phone rings, stay where you are, consciously breathe in and out, and smile to yourself. Repeat for the second ring. Then consciously, slowly, pick up the phone on the third ring. "You can afford to practice breathing and smiling like this, because if the person has something important to say, she will certainly wait for at least three rings," writes the Buddhist monk in *Peace Is Every Step*. "You know that you are smiling not only for your own sake, but also for the sake of the other person. If you are irritated or angry, the other person will receive your negativity. But because you have been breathing consciously and smiling, you are dwelling in mindfulness, and when you pick up the phone, how fortunate for the person calling you!"

This works the other way too. Practice taking three conscious breaths and smiling to yourself before you make a call, and you'll be more collected and happy before you begin speaking.

Create a Heart Connection

As a child and a young woman, I lived by my head. And I still don't knock it—my mind has served me well over the years. But as I get older, more and more what matters to me, what brings me joy, is not the stunning brilliance of a person's mind, but their ability to create a heartfelt connection. And for myself, I've ceased asking, How smart can I be? and have begun to ask, How kind can I be? How compassionate? How loving? I guess it's because I've become convinced, as my friend Daphne Rose Kingma says so eloquently in her book *True Love*, "In the end, nothing we do or say in this lifetime will matter as much as the way we have loved one another."

And I want my loving to go far and wide, to encompass not only those who are the dearest to me, but my deaf neighbor, the coworker I struggle with, and you, the reader. So that's why I love the following practice I found in Nancy Napier's book, *Sacred Practices for Conscious Living*. Today, whenever you interact with someone, or even if you just think of a person, "imagine that you are linked to them with a line of light, heart-to-heart." Visualize a beam of light flowing from you to the other person, and from her or him back to you. Notice what changes as a consequence of the heart connection.

Get into Hot Water

Remember Fizzies? You'd drop tablets in a glass of water, and soon you would have a bubbly fruit drink. Well, now someone has invented some for the bathtub. Drop one in your tub and watch the fizzy bubbles rise. The secret ingredient? Baking soda, which happens to be good for your skin as well as fun in the tub. Brand names include Bath Fizzies, Bath Bombs, Get Fresh!, and Bath Bloomers Botanical Pollens.

Put Your Woes in a Drawer and Close it

Our minds, left to their own devices, are unruly creatures. They wander all over or get stuck thinking about the same things over and over. Stop obsessing about a problem you can't fix. Much of what worries us is just not fixable.

Here's a trick to try. When you find yourself obsessing about something, write it down on a piece of paper, stick it in a drawer, and close it. Tell yourself that you can open the drawer tomorrow and read it again, but between now and then, it's off limits. Who knows? By tomorrow, the problem may have gone away on its own or you may have some up with a solution.

Get High on GABA

Many alternative health experts sing the praises of GABA (gamma-amino butyric acid), claiming it to be the perfect natural tranquilizer. If you suffer from depression, you might want to give it a try. The recommended dosage is 2,000 mg a day; it is available at health food stores and nutrition centers.

Pat a Pet

Pets are great happiness boosters. The companionship, love, and entertainment a pet provides is, for many people, as significant as any human relationship.

You don't even have to own a pet. Researchers tell us that touching, holding, patting, or even just looking at an animal lowers blood pressure and makes us feel better. Many hospitals and nursing homes now have programs to take advantage of these healing effects.

So stroke your cat, hug the dog, or borrow a neighbor's pet for a good pat, and you'll be happier and healthier for it.

Have Something to Look Forward To

We all need something pulling us into the future—a dream that we want to make come true, that gives us the incentive to get up in the morning. When my sister turned thirty-nine, she found herself depressed. It took her a while to figure out why: "I had spent the last ten years of my life focused on three things—having a good relationship, creating a family, and buying a house. Now I've done them all, and there's nothing left on my list!" She had everything she wanted, but because she had nothing to look forward to, she was unhappy.

So make a "want to do" list. It doesn't have to be as ambitious as my sister's. Just anything that you want to accomplish: create a beautiful garden, go to Costa Rica, learn to play the saxophone, hang glide. Simply creating the list will help you make your dream come true.

Give Up Magical Thinking

Deep in my heart I believe that if I worry about something, I will prevent it from happening—if I worry about the plane my husband is on crashing, I will keep it in the air. If I worry about my stepdaughter driving late at night, she'll arrive home safely. But the more I worry, the less happy I am in any given moment.

In truth, worry is *not* preparation, nor is it a magic pill that prevents things from occurring. The plane will crash or not (most likely not) whether you worry or not. Your company will have layoffs or not, regardless of your worrying. Our lack of control over what happens is why we worry in the first place. One thing I've found to be helpful when I find myself worrying is to acknowledge that I feel out of control and to ask what I can do about the situation to prepare for whatever I am envisioning. Maybe there is an action I *can* take—dust off the résumé, talk to others who have dealt with the problem, have the mole I'm worrying about checked out—and maybe all I can do is recognize that it is out of my control and send up a silent prayer that all will turn out well.

Hug This Moment

Sarah Quigley, in *Facing Fear, Finding Courage,* suggests that we "hug *this* moment, not the one ahead that you hope will be different. Encircle it with a thank-you, even if tears are in your eyes and despair is in your heart. It is the one sure way that life is guaranteed to be better no matter what your circumstances."

APRIL
18

Clean Out the Closet

When I was working on the book *Simple Pleasures,* a collection of stories about the little things that bring people happiness, I was struck by how many folks mentioned cleaning—laundry, vacuuming, straightening up a desk, bringing order to a coat closet. The miracle of turning chaos or filth into beauty and cleanliness truly is one of life's small satisfactions, particularly when it is not compulsory.

Where can you bring a little order or beauty right now? Throwing out that pile of magazines that has accumulated next to your desk? Finally finding storage space for all the items that have been cluttering your kitchen counter? Pick one area that has been driving you crazy and bring a little order to it. You'll feel great.

Bottom's Up

After a long hard, winter, Vermonters swear by this pick-me-up. It's said to increase energy, particularly if you feel fatigued as soon as you wake up in the morning.

Combine 1 teaspoon honey, 2 tablespoons apple cider vinegar, and 1 cup warm water in a blender. Stir thoroughly. Sure to wake you up.

Reframe Failure

One of the greatest creative geniuses of the twentieth century was Thomas Edison, who spent years trying to generate electricity. Before he made his discovery, he was asked about all his "failures." He replied, "I have not failed. I have found thousands of ways that will not produce electric light. I am that much closer to discovering one that will."

What an attitude! It not only allowed him to keep on going so that he ultimately did discover how to generate electricity, but it kept him happy as he went about the process.

Is there something going on in your life that could use this kind of reframing? When I met my husband-to-be, he had never had a relationship that lasted longer than six months. When I asked him about it, he said that whenever a relationship ended, he always told himself that he still needed to learn more. Learn he did—we've now been together seven years.

Drop Your Expectations

Don't go around saying the world owes you a living;
the world owes you nothing; it was here first.
—Mark Twain

When I was thinking about and writing a book on gratitude, it struck me that expectations are the murderers of gratefulness and happiness. When we expect something, if it arrives, we tend to take it for granted; after all, we believed we deserved it and were counting on it happening. And if what we expect doesn't arrive, we have a tendency to wallow in resentment and self-pity. After all, we deserved it, so why didn't we get it? The world must be out to get us.

The happiest people I know are those who live without expectations. As a consequence, they are able to appreciate all the wonderful big and little things that come their way and are less miserable when things go wrong.

How have expectations stood in your way? Expectations about how a relationship should be? What kind of gifts you should receive? How your family should interact? Drop your expectations and you will be emotionally available to whatever great things come your way.

Indulge Your Innocent Craving

I have a confession to make—I love Coca-Cola. As in six-cans-a-day-if-I-didn't-control-myself love. For years after my college Coke bingeing, I resisted altogether. Never bought it, never drank it. Then I married someone with the same secret passion, and it crept back into the house. I wavered, worried, and finally decided that I could enjoy one Coke per day maximum, no more. And I've kept to my commitment for years. Many days I have none, but when I do choose to have one, I really enjoy it. I drink it consciously, noticing the bubbles as it goes down my throat, the cold sweetness on my tongue. I savor my Coke, wringing every drop of pleasure out of those 140 calories.

Just for today, indulge your innocent craving (this is not permission for alcoholics to drink, food addicts to eat or ex-pot heads to smoke; I'm talking harmless nonaddictive pleasures)—the Chunky Monkey ice cream; the chocolate cake with mocha frosting; the bananas with peanut butter. Whatever it is that you love to eat but avoid because you are being good. Go ahead and splurge. And while you're splurging, really relish it. That way it will be less likely to become habit-forming.

Surprise Someone

My stepdaughter recently went to Europe. While she was in the bathroom just before leaving, I snuck $100 in her backpack with a card saying it was "splurge" money. I had such fun—thinking of the idea, finding the perfect hiding place, trying not to get caught. It was so fun that it didn't even matter to me if she appreciated it or not! (She did, days later, when rooting around in her pack.)

Put a little lift in your life and surprise someone you know.

Write Yourself a Love Letter

You've grown a lot in your life. Only you really know how far you've come, the progress you've made. Reflect right now on the positive changes you can see in yourself and write a short note of appreciation to yourself for all that you've learned. Be specific as possible—you've done a great job of learning to listen to others, you've excelled at looking on the bright side—and be your own secret admirer.

Root Out Happiness Suppressers

Recently I realized that whenever someone asked me how I was, I would say, "OK," rather than "Great," or even, "Fine." When I thought about it, I saw that I was afraid of sounding too happy—afraid to make the other person feel bad in comparison (!), but more important, afraid to "jinx" myself (you know—once the powers that be hear that you're happy, they'll send a plague of locusts to put you in your place).

What screwy thinking! The truth is, happiness is contagious. The more I am happy, the more you will feel happy in my presence. And there is no evil spirit lurking around ready to put us in our place if we feel too happy. What stories are you telling yourself to keep you from feeling as happy as you can? Take a few moments to think about them.

Once I realized what I was doing, I vowed to say, "Great" when asked how I was. I have not been completely successful (old habits die hard), but I'm trying.

Feed Your Mind Well

When I was in therapy, I used to drag myself into my therapist's office every week, mildly depressed. One day, she asked me what I had been reading, and I replied, "The biography of Sylvia Plath" (the famous poet who killed herself). "Stop," she said. "Her unhappiness is making you miserable." Then she gave me an inspiring book about women who thrived against great odds in the American West in the 1800s. I must admit it did make me feel better.

It's true that misery loves company, and so does happiness. You can elevate your spirits through your choice of reading material. An uplifting book of quotes, a wonderful novel, *Hope* magazine. Feed your mind positive images, and you'll feel better.

Try Bach Flower Remedies

These are thirty-eight flower essences developed in the 1930s by Edward Bach, a homeopath who believed that negative emotional states caused illness and prevented healing. He claimed that to heal and be healthy, you need to be happy. So he created these remedies to relieve mental distress and consequently promote healing. Like all homeopathic remedies, they are dilutions of substances that work on the energetic body (the electromagnetic field that surrounds the physical body and every living cell). Believers claim that the essence of the plant's property remains in the dilution and that those properties can stabilize emotional sensitivities.

You select the appropriate remedy based on personality. Here are a few: Gentian for those who are easily discouraged, cry or give up; Willow for those who feel they are being picked on or life is unfair; Pine for those who are stuck in self-blame and self-criticism; Impatiens for those who are impatient or tense; Rose for gloominess; Gorse for despair and hopelessness. I'm going to give Impatiens a try.

Let Go of That
Which You Can't Control

Stoic philosopher Epictetus was a former Roman slave who wrote a great deal about personal happiness. His primary tenet was to know what you can and cannot control. Those things you can control, you should; those you can't should be released. "Within our control," he wrote, "are our own opinions, aspirations, desires, and the things that repel us. . . . Outside our control, however, are such things as what kind of body we have, whether we're born into wealth or strike it rich, how we are regarded by others, and our status in society. We must remember that those things are externals and are therefore not our concern."

I don't know about you, but I sure try to control all kinds of things—not only in my own life but in other people's. My desire for control gets out of control particularly when it comes to other people's feelings—I try to manage so-and-so's reaction to a third party, to finesse so-and-so's response to something. It's exhausting—and useless.

What do you try to control? Money? People's image of you? The circumstances of life? Just notice where you are a control freak and see if you can loosen your grip just a little. Life has a way of being messy and un-nail-downable; people do and feel what they want independently of you.

Get Out in the Sun

We all know the dangers of too much sun exposure. But did you know that a moderate amount of sunlight, particularly morning sun, is good for you? Many of us are aware that our bodies create vitamin D from sunlight, but recent research shows that a half-hour of sun in the morning will elevate our mood and energy. That's because, according to Norma Rosenthal, M.D., author of *Winter Blues,* "Sunlight increases the production of serotonin and norepinephrine," which are natural uppers. And why morning light? "In the morning," says the good doctor, "the eyes are most sensitive to the mood-altering effects of light."

So put on some sunscreen and get out in the morning sun. You'll not only feel better, but you'll sleep better too. Regular exposure to morning sun helps keep your body's internal clock ticking on schedule.

Give a May Basket

When I was a kid, we always made May baskets for all the houses in our neighborhood to celebrate May Day. We would get such a thrill out of making them, hanging them on front doorknobs, and then ringing the bell and running to a hiding spot where we'd watch the faces of the recipients.

May baskets are incredibly easy to make. All you need are some flowers (we always picked the first wildflowers of the season, but storebought is OK) that you've fashioned into an attractive bouquet tied with a rubber band and placed in a cone basket. To make the cone, take an 8½ by 11-inch piece of construction paper rolled into a ice-cream cone shape, with the top wider than the bottom. Staple into place and attach a paper handle (a ½-inch-wide strip of construction paper) at the top with staples.

Whose day can you brighten with such a gift? Your coworkers? The neighbors? Your daughter?

Practice Mindful Homecoming

This is a wonderful idea from Lama Surya Das' book *Awakening to the Sacred*. We tend to run in the door at the end of the day, bringing all our issues and problems with us. Tonight, try something different and notice the effect it has on you and your family.

"When you return home, rejoice. Stand in front of your door and appreciate the moment of your arrival. Breathe in and out three times. Mark the passage and completeness of the circle [of coming and going]. Feel the satisfaction. Just be there for a moment. Now open the door and step inside. Home is a temple; your sacred domain. Come home to yourself. Oh, and don't forget to be mindful of where you place your keys. You will want them for further journeying."

Take Money Out of the Equation

No matter how many times I write about it, deep in the recesses of my reptilian brain, I still continue to believe that money could make me happy. So any time I find something to help me get over that misconception, I jump on it.

In his book *Baby Steps to Happiness,* John Q. Baucom reminds us that money doesn't buy happiness. He uses the metaphor of oxygen: "In its absence, money is like a lack of oxygen. It can create serious problems. But in its presence, money is like oxygen as well. Just because you breathe doesn't mean you're happy."

Easy to say, right? But here's a way to take money out the picture altogether and focus on what might really make you happy. It's a technique from Jonathan Robinson's *Shortcuts to Bliss.* Write down what you would do if you had $1 billion. Now, imagine that you still have the $1 billion but that you were required by law to work forty hours a week. What would you do? "In other words, what is work that you find so rewarding that you would do it for free?" Your answer is an important clue as to what would make you happiest.

Create a Happiness List

What makes you happy? It's different for each of us. Here is my friend Pat's list: When I really feel listened to; when I have the bed all to myself; when I take a hot bubble bath; when my son Khari gives me a big hug and holds on tight.

Make your own list.

Get Up with Gingko

Gingko biloba is an herb that is known for improving memory, but studies have indicated that it's a great anti-anxiety agent as well. According to Harold H. Bloomfield, M.D., author of *Healing Anxiety with Herbs,* 120 to 180 mg a day lowers anxiety by as much as 79 percent. This is accomplished by increasing bloodflow to the brain, which heightens the amount of dopamine in the bloodstream. Dopamine is a brain chemical that enhances calm thinking under stress. Gingko is available at health food stores and nutrition centers.

Call In Well

At my office we have one day a month to use as we want—for sick days, Grandma in town days, just don't feel like coming in days. I consider it to be a good mental health policy—I don't want people working if they don't want to be there, and I want to discourage lying. Why must you pretend you are sick if you want to play hooky with your kids or spouse?

Take the day and do something fun.

Relax

Here's a wonderful relaxation technique you can do before going to sleep or any time you need a de-stressor. Light a candle and sit in comfortable position in a dark room. Look at the candle while consciously relaxing each part of your body. Begin with your toes. Tighten them for a moment, and then let go. Move to your foot, your calf, your thighs, tightening each and then releasing while watching the candle. Move to your buttocks, your lower back, your stomach, and chest. Tighten and relax your upper back, neck, and shoulders, your arms and hands, your face, your mouth, your eyes, your forehead. Blow out the candle and go to sleep.

Have a Chocolate Bar

The more I try to deprive myself of food indulgences, the more weight I gain and the crabbier I am. Women in particular tend to crave chocolate, particularly when premenstrual, and there's a good reason for it. Chocolate contains mood-lifting chemicals such as theobromine, and increases endorphins and serotonin in the blood, which promote euphoria and calm. According to Aztec legend, cacao seeds come from Paradise, and eating them brings wisdom and power.

So today, give yourself a chocolate treat and notice the effect. After you indulge, don't scold yourself. Study after study has shown that moderate amounts of treats are better than complete deprivation (which tends to lead to bingeing). And remember, what you eat over the course of a week matters more than any one given day. Strive for balance, not perfection.

Practice Random Acts of Kindness™

When we at Conari Press published the first *Random Acts of Kindness*™ book, we knew it would help people be more kind in their lives. But we had no idea the notion would so captivate people. Inundated with mail from people telling their stories, we have gone on to create a Random Acts of Kindness™ week, a foundation, and now a worldwide Kindness Day, the first of which will be celebrated in November 2000.

The reason for this groundswell of support is that doing acts of kindness for no reason makes us feel good. It reaffirms our connection with one another and adds to the light in the world. And they are so easy to do—putting a quarter in a stranger's parking meter takes less than a minute, but gives a great burst of joy.

So today, be a kindness angel and do something nice for a stranger.

Give Yourself Permission
to Be Yourself

Today is the day to be kind to ourselves. It's OK to be you, just as you are. As old, as fat, as lazy, or as tired as you may be. The amount of psychic energy you'll free up from obsessing about yourself will make it possible to feel happy in the present moment.

Tricks for Stress

When you have a lot to do, you can begin to feel overwhelmed, spiraling down into lethargy. In this state, you feel you have so much to do that you can't do anything at all. Try to break what you need to do into small steps. Make a list of everything you have to do. Then take care of the easiest items on the list. You'll stop the cycle of helplessness and give yourself a boost in the right direction.

Or perhaps the sense of having too much to do makes you speed around like a maniac, doing a bit of everything but getting nothing done completely or well. When I find myself in this place, I've learned to say to myself: I have all the time I need to do this. It really works! Somehow the mental ease it creates makes it possible for me to do whatever is needed in a timely yet non-rushed fashion.

Take a "Gratitude Moment"

This is the easiest and quickest happiness enhancer I know. Take a deep breath and think of three things you are grateful for, right in this moment.

MAY

12

Go on a Mental Vacation

In a tape on worry, Earl Nightingale claimed we spend time worrying this way: 40 percent on things that never happen; 30 percent on things that have already happened that can't be changed; 12 percent on needless worries about our health, 10 percent on miscellaneous needless worries; and only 8 percent on worries that are legitimate.

So much of what I put my daily thoughts and energy toward are worrying about things that never come to pass. What if, instead, I thought more like Scarlett O'Hara in *Gone with the Wind:* "I'll think about that tomorrow." This is a great happiness technique when dealing with something over which you have no control. Won't work forever, but try going worry-free for today.

Create a Fan Club

Make a list of the friends who boost you up. You know, the ones you can call any time of the day or night and know that they will bring a smile to your face. Then don't be afraid to use your list when you need it. It's OK to ask for support.

Look around You

Notice one thing in your natural environment today that brings a lift to your heart. For me it is discovering that the California Pepperwood trees in my new house bloom in the spring with white flowers that look and smell very much like wisteria. I moved here in the summer and saw them drop their leaves, transforming the side of my house into a barren winterland, then bud and leaf in the early spring. Now in May, they are in full bloom with pendulant white blossoms that fill the air with fragrance. An incredible surprise!

What will you discover?

Take a Dip in the Ocean—At Home

Have you ever noticed how great you feel after a swim in the ocean? Part of the reason is that the magnesium, zinc, and potassium in sea salt draws out the lactic acid from your muscles, easing tension. You can simulate the effect in a luxurious bath. Pour 1 cup of salt into the stream of warm water while filling the tub, turn on an ocean surf CD or tape, light a seabreeze-scented candle, and indulge.

Check Out These
Herbal Sleep Remedies

If you have been suffering from insomnia and the other remedies in this book aren't working, try lemon balm (official name *Melissa officinalis*). According to the German government, it's a great sleep inducer that has no known side effects. It works by soothing anxiety that may be causing sleeplessness. Just before bed, brew up a cup. Put 2 to 4 teaspoons of the dried herb (available at herb stores or you can grow it easily yourself) in a cup of boiling water. You can also take it in capsule form; look for lemon balm in health food stores or nutrition centers.

Chamomile, hops, and evening primrose are also known to help with insomnia. They too can be brewed into teas or taken as supplements. Follow label instructions.

Smile Just for Today

A smile is a light on your face that lets people know your heart is home.
—Anonymous

Today, make a commitment to yourself to smile at everyone who crosses your path: the crabby check-out clerk, your harried boss, and notice what effect it has on them—and you! It's almost impossible to smile at someone and not have them smile back.

You don't even have to feel like it. Researchers have discovered that smiling is so powerful a happiness booster that our mood improves any time we turn up the corners of our mouth—even if it is only to hold a pen between our teeth.

Dance Away

Research has shown that having fun is one of the best stress busters in the world. You don't even have to leave the house. Just put on your favorite music and shake your body. I like to dance with my two-year-old. Watching her moves makes me laugh, and I don't even notice that I am actually getting exercise.

Dancing has other benefits. It integrates the right and left hemispheres of the brain (a good thing when you do work that is mostly one side or the other), and when you dance with a partner, you bolster your immune system by eliminating feelings of loneliness (a sense of isolation can lead to disease).

Many of us don't want to dance, because we're afraid of looking foolish, of not knowing the right moves. The remedy? Do it alone, with no one watching, as an experiment in goal-lessness. Try not to judge yourself (or just acknowledge your judgment as it arises and let it drift away). Maybe closing your eyes will help; maybe not. But try it and see how you feel.

Declare a Watchless Day

Take off your timepiece today and go at your own rhythm. As Jean Shinoda Bolen says in *Crossing to Avalon*, "In the rigorously scheduled, productive . . . world measured by Father Time, we suffer the lack of the kind of nourishing activities in which we lose track of time—when we can play or just enjoy being instead of doing. A flat, dry depression results; there are no tears or grief; existence is joyless."

Break Your Routine

Most of us live such routine-bound lives—the nine-to-five grind, the two-hour commute, the errands on the weekend we can't do any other time. Routine leads to passivity; we fall asleep to our own lives. I noticed this recently as I backed out of my driveway on my way to work. So used to doing it, I wasn't even looking and I barely missed a car that was parked in a different (non-routine) spot.

Paradoxically, most of us are so busy that we have to schedule in spontaneity. I'm suggesting that today, after reading this, you do something out of the ordinary. Stay in bed late, climb a mountain—whatever breaks the pattern of your life—and notice how much more alive, vibrant, and refreshed you feel.

Renew Your Energy in a Flash

Herbalists are singing the praises of a new energy booster—Arctic root (*Rhodiola rosea*), which is said to increase energy four times better than ginseng. (It also strengthens your heart.) A 100-mg dose goes to work in less than an hour, boosting stamina, mental capacity, and muscle strength. Consult a doctor before taking it if you have any health conditions, and be sure to follow label directions.

Set a Goal That Matters to You

Researchers at the University of Miami have discovered something that should have been obvious. If a particular goal doesn't matter to us intrinsically (we're working toward something solely to win praise or acceptance, not to satisfy a true inner longing), then reaching it does not bring us happiness.

Think about your current goals. Do they come from an inner desire? Or are they to please others or gain social acceptance? Are they someone else's ideas of what you should be doing? True happiness comes from achieving a goal that we care about, regardless of what anyone else thinks. Pick one goal today that matters to you alone.

Do Something Nice
for Someone You Love

I asked my husband recently what makes him happy. One of his first responses was, "Bringing you flowers for no reason." He's in touch with that happiness that comes from bringing someone else pleasure, and we can all tap into that automatic feel-good.

It doesn't matter whom you choose or what you do to please them. Just that you do it.

The Purpose of Fear

When I think about my life as a whole, I would say fear is my greatest obstacle to happiness. My fears are many: I fear losing the people I love; I fear my ability to support myself; I fear the state of the world and the future.

Because I know that fear inhibits happiness, I'm ever alert to techniques to deal effectively with fear. Here's one I have found particularly insightful from Robin Lysne: Take a piece of paper and make two columns vertically. In the left-hand column, write down all your fears. In the right-hand column, write down what purpose each fear serves in your life. What did you discover?

When I looked at my lists overall, I learned that my fears are a way of trying to control the future, because I confuse planning with worrying. How about you?

Take a Mental Sabbatical

Pretend you are taking a year off. Make a list of what you would do, then figure out how to make at least one thing on your list come true.

Root Out Your Negative Self-Talk

What are the negative messages you've incorporated as part of your self-talk? Some common ones are "No pain, no gain"; "Life is a struggle and then you die"; "Watch out for the other guy." Mine was that it is noble to suffer—and as a consequence, I've had plenty of suffering.

Because we, at least in part, create our reality through how we talk to ourselves, it's important if we want to be happy to make sure we're not bringing ourselves down with negative messages, but instead raising our spirits through positive ones. Think about the negative messages you've absorbed about life. What positive thing could you say to yourself instead? My substitute' for "'Tis noble to suffer" is "It's OK if it's easy."

Stop Living in the Past

When I look over my life, I see that I've spent a good deal of time thinking about happiness I've experienced in the past and mourning its loss. I spent fourteen years lamenting the end of a seven-year relationship, which did nothing for my ability to be happy in the relationship I was currently in. And, when I was honest with myself, my trips down memory lane were less than accurate. Like anyone wallowing in nostalgia, I remembered only the good things, and ignored all the pain and difficulties that were also present. I painted the past in a rosy glow and then bemoaned its loss.

Does this sound familiar? Or perhaps you do something slightly different—maybe you try to recreate times that you were happy—the trip to the Bahamas, the picnic by the lake—and are frustrated when you don't have the same feelings about the experience. That's because nothing can ever be exactly the same, if only because we've already experienced it, and we make ourselves miserable when we try.

Right now, examine the ways you keep yourself from happiness now by living in the past, and commit to coming into the present, with all the potential for happiness that it holds.

Find Something Orange

Color therapy is the use of colors to promote emotional well-being. It has been used throughout history to influence moods and in recent decades, psychologists have devised tests to demonstrate that color does influence how we feel (and even how fast we eat, hence the bright colors of fast food restaurants, designed to get you out the door quickly). For example, the Blackfriars Lodge in London, which was painted black, was known for a high suicide rate. When the building was painted green, the rate dropped by one-third.

So, to enhance happiness, avoid black, violet, and blue (all can increase depression). What colors should you surround yourself with? According to color therapists: orange. Orange promotes optimism, enthusiasm, and happiness. Red also can help overcome depression but is not recommended for overly excitable personalities.

So buy an orange flower today, use an orange-colored light in your living room, or put a big bowl of oranges in your office, and see if you feel happier.

Do a Freeze Frame

This is a technique to combat anxiety, fear, or anger developed by HeartMath, a California research institute. It comes from research that shows that feeling love and appreciation produces a smooth heart rhythm, which positively affects the body's immune, neurological, and endocrine systems, and creates a sense of happiness and well-being.

It has five steps:

1. When you first notice yourself having a negative feeling, "freeze-frame" it. Stop, as if pushing the pause button on a VCR.

2. Move your awareness to your heart. For ten seconds, imagine breathing through your heart.

3. For another ten seconds, bring to mind a person, place, or thing that you love and feel your feelings of love.

4. Ask your heart how best to respond to the situation that is causing you anxiety or anger.

5. Do what your heart tells you.

Stop Rescuing

If someone in my general vicinity is unhappy, I feel immediate panic. Are they unhappy with me? Even if the answer is no, I feel compelled to try and fix the situation. Sound familiar?

As Iyanla Vanzant and many other teachers have said, "People learn what they need to learn the way they choose to learn it, and there is nothing we can do about their choice." We can offer a kind word, a willing ear, but they are going to make their own choices.

If this is an issue for you too, you might want to try some of the phrases I've taught myself. I say to myself, "This is not your issue, this is theirs." When appropriate, I say to the other person, "I am sorry you are suffering. How can I support you?" That way, if there is some way I can be helpful, they will tell me. Otherwise I can let it go.

Avoid the Low-Blood-Sugar Blues

If you find yourself irritable and unable to think clearly when you get too hungry, you may be suffering from low blood sugar. Ironically, it is often caused by high sugar intake. In response to large amounts of sugar, the pancreas releases extra insulin, which lowers your blood sugar, making you blue. To even yourself out, go for small, well-balanced, low-sugar meals, as frequently as six times a day.

Hide a Love Note

I have a friend who has had a troubled relationship with her father. But no matter how difficult things between them get, she always remembers that when she was in junior high and high school, after her mother had abandoned the family, her father would often put in her backpack a love note that she would see as she took her books out at school. Those notes not only created joy in the moment, but also now, years later.

Who in your life would be delighted to receive a surprise love note? Tuck one in a child's lunch box, a spouse's brief case, under a pillow. You'll increase happiness for both of you.

Identify Local Flora and Fauna

I recently moved to a house on a creek, and one of the joys of living there has been learning about the birds that live nearby or migrate through. I bought an inexpensive guidebook and have begun to pull it out whenever a bird I don't recognize flies by.

When we know the names of the birds, trees, and flowers in our environment, we create a more intimate relationship with them. We feel more connected to nature, and to the great wheel of life. From that connection comes a satisfying sense of belonging.

Today, pledge to learn the name of one plant, tree, or bird in your environment. If you don't have a guidebook, ask a coworker about the bush outside the office door; your neighbor about the flowers in her front yard. Notice how it makes you feel.

Wake Up Differently

If you're like me, chances are you wake up thinking about all you have to do today—the schedule of meetings, the projects that must get done, the problems to be confronted. Then we add to the mental weight load by worrying about them all.

Today, try something different. When you awaken, focus on how you want to be as you go through your day, rather than what you have to do. You might say something like, "As I go through today, I choose to be kind and patient to myself and others." When I have to do publicity, which makes me nervous, I say, "May what I have to say serve the common good." By setting an intention—kindness, patience, service—we bring more of our essence to any encounter, and focus on the positive that we can do, no matter what else is going on.

Do One Little Thing That's Been Nagging at You

Procrastination is a giant happiness killer. We can't fully appreciate the present moment when in the back of our minds we're thinking about all the things we have to do that we've been avoiding. Usually, it takes less energy to actually do whatever it is than not to do it.

The piles of files in your office, the fountain you've been meaning to put up on the wall for months, the letter you need to write. Pick one nagging little thing and do it today. Doesn't that feel absolutely great?

Take a Love Inventory

Perhaps great love is not a person but all of life lived fully,
all the love encountered along the way. . . .
—Misty Santana

I love this thought, probably because it matches perfectly my life experience.

Take a few moments right now to think about all the ways you have been loved in your life. It may not have come in the ways you expected or imagined, it may not have lasted as long as you wished, but you have been loved by many people.

Visualize Contentment

It's so easy to fall into the "if only" trap. You know, the one in which happiness is just around the corner if only a certain thing happened: I would be happy if only my retirement account was bigger, if my child were doing well in school, if I had the relationship I desired. . . .

What a set-up for perpetual misery. You'll be unhappy if these things never come to pass, and you won't even be happy if they do (because you've expected them to carry too much meaning). Happiness only comes from choosing to be happy, no matter what our circumstances. A friend reminded me of that recently. She said, "I was in a relationship for fourteen years with one person and was unhappy, believing that if only my partner were different I would be happy. Now I am in a relationship with someone completely different and am still unhappy. Obviously it has nothing to do with my relationship!"

Here's a practice to help you stop doing "if only." When you find yourself saying, "If only," imagine putting those words in a hot air balloon and visualize the balloon floating up into space.

Live with Your Poisonous Trees

In her book *Voices from the Heart,* Christina Feldman writes of visiting a paradisiacal tropical island that seemed to have no flaws. Except one. On the island in several public places grew some poisonous trees; one drop of sap on the skin could send a person into shock. Visitors were warned of them, but Christina asked an islander, "If they are so dangerous, why haven't they been cut down?"

"Why would we do that?" the man replied. "They were here before we were, and they are part of the landscape of our island. It is up to us to take care around them."

The incident struck her because it is such a powerful analogy for how we need to relate to the world. "Many of us have poisonous trees in our lives. . . . We have relationships with people who are difficult. And sometimes we carry these poisonous trees within ourselves—in our behavior patterns, fears, or habitual reactions. . . . Can we simply acknowledge and accept them? Can we treat them with respect, care, and understanding? Do we recognize that they are part of our personal landscape? Or do we try to eliminate them?"

We can never eliminate all the poisonous trees in our lives. It's just not possible. Take a few minutes today to think about what changing your attitude about the poisonous trees in your life would do for your happiness.

Do an Office Check

We spend so much time at work, and poorly lit or ventilated offices can really sap our energy and make us feel sluggish and depressed. The best offices have plenty of fresh air and natural light. If you are stuck with fluorescent lights, consider buying full-spectrum bulbs—they're expensive but worth it. They fix into the fluorescent fixtures and simulate natural light. Especially important for light-sensitive folks.

If your office is uncheery and the company allows for creativity, consider a cubicle beautification program. One of my coworkers who has no exterior window had a friend paint one wall with sky. Another made a fountain for her desk. Bring in plants, artwork, or photographs from home.

When considering paint colors, be aware that scientists tell us the most soothing colors are pink and blue, but do what feels right to you. (I hate pink and blue.)

Toast Yourself

My two-year-old has started a wonderful tradition in our house. Little ones are great mimics, and Ana is no exception. Months ago, we had friends over for dinner and someone gave a toast. Now, every evening as we sit down to dinner, Ana picks up her glass of juice and says, "Toast!" The three of us clink glasses and I say, "To love and being together." It's a marvelous moment in the day.

You can incorporate this into your own life in many ways. You can give a silent toast to yourself—after all, you're worth it. Or you can say something to those with whom you live. If you are uncomfortable being spontaneous, you could memorize a moving toast and give it tonight or on a special occasion. Check out *Toasts* by Paul Dickson.

Practice SAFE

This is a technique for developing what Paul Pearsall calls our "Seventh Sense," the part of ourselves that feeds our soul by connecting to what gives us joy. He calls it "SAFE": Sit and Feel Everything. All you do is sit down quietly, in a natural place, if possible, and notice what you are feeling. Not what you are thinking, but what you feel. Notice your bottom on the chair, the feel of the sun on your face. Notice too what emotions come up for you. Whatever you are experiencing is all right. Look at the natural world around you and feel your connection to it and those you love. SAFE is not a meditation practice, says Pearsall, but a "fascination" one.

Pearsall makes big claims for SAFE. "Most of us who practice it regularly notice that just doing nothing and feeling everything tends to produce powerful results," he writes in *Write Your Own Pleasure Prescription*. "You will likely notice that your SAFE period is followed by receipt of good news, the resolution of a problem you may have experienced, or the emergence of new life possibilities." Sounds good to me.

Play with Paint

Or crayons or pastels or any other drawing medium. This is about drawing what you feel inside by creating an energy or mood painting. I like to do it first thing on awakening in the morning. Place a pad of paper and crayons next to the bed. As soon as you wake, before your mind is fully engaged and when your last dream is still with you, lean over, pick up paper and colors, and draw how you feel. It doesn't have to look like anything—in fact it shouldn't. It should just be an abstract expression of your feelings.

You can do this anytime. With your children or mate when you are feeling annoyed at one another and words would just make it worse. When you feel particularly happy. Or sad. Or hopeless or full of energy. It's a visual representation of your feelings and as such, should never be judged or interpreted by anyone, including yourself. Just draw or paint and let yourself experience the joy that comes from putting down your feelings on paper, as if you were an uninhibited preschooler again.

Boost Your Energy

In her book *Natural Energy,* Dr. Erika Schwartz cites compelling medical evidence from the United States and abroad for taking two supplements daily: L-carnitine and Coenzyme Q-10 (CoQ10). They offer a number of health benefits, ranging from helping chronic fatigue syndrome to heart disease and infertility. Carnitine in particular, she writes, is a "powerful natural mood elevator that can help relieve the toxic effect of living in a highly stressful world." Patients taking both, she claims, report more energy and less fatigue, elevated mood, and sense of well-being. Many of her patients were able to stop taking antidepressants after taking these supplements for only four weeks.

Her recommendation for the average person? 500 mg of carnitine and 30 mg of CoQ10 with breakfast and the same with lunch. Don't take these if you are undergoing radiation, and be sure to always take them with a full glass of water. Do not take on an empty stomach. For a full explanation and suggestions for particular problems, consult Dr. Schwartz's book.

Fall Madly in Love with the World

Ruth Bernard is a renowned photographer with an incredible passion for living. At age eighty-one, with two artificial knees, she climbed Mt. Fuji in Japan. "It looked so shiny and beautiful from the train there was nothing to do—I had to climb it."

Recently she was asked for her recipe for a long and happy life. Among her suggestions was the thought for this day. How do you fall in love with the world? Just like with a human being. By noticing and appreciating all its little peculiarities and idiosyncrasies—the way the clouds float by, the play of light on dark green pine needles, the kiss of the wind on your skin.

Today, take a few moments to "fall in love" with the world around you.

Find Your Oracle

An oracle is a messenger who delivers a prophecy. The Greek Oracle at Delphi is probably the best known. But oracles abound; life is full of signs for us to interpret.

There is a wonderful message for you today in nature. It is in the wind, or a bird, a tree, the dragonfly that floats past, the way the afternoon light slants into your bedroom—some aspect of nature. Pay attention to what is an oracle for you today and discover the message. It will make you smile.

Tell Your Story

Telling your story is healing, and others are healed by hearing it, if only that they find the courage to tell theirs. This is so true that psychologists have recently discovered that when survivors of the recent wars in Eastern Europe told their stories (accounts of rape, genocide, and other horrors), their symptoms of Post-Traumatic Stress Disorder—anger, nightmares, depression, and violence—dropped 25 percent, and six months later, 47 percent had no symptoms of PTSD. Said one survivor, "When I speak to someone who listens to me, and who respects me, I feel good." What's your story?

Pick Your Mood

Different scents induce different moods. Here are a variety of essential oils known to relieve depression and increase happiness: chamomile, clary sage, geranium, lemon, patchouli, rose, rosewood, ylang ylang. Why not experiment to find one you really like? You can use it in body lotion, bathwater, or massage oil; apply directly to pulse points; or combine with water and put in an atomizer for a skin or air refresher. Be careful: If you have sensitive skin, undiluted oils can cause allergic reactions.

Expand Your Mind

Some of our unhappiness, I'm convinced, comes from boredom. Our minds get stuck in ruts, particularly if we're not learning something new.

One of the ways my coworker Brenda keeps her mind vibrant is by subscribing to an e-mail service that sends you a word a day. "It never fails to bring a smile to my face," she says. Today's word is *longnimity* (long-guy-NIM-i-tee), which means calmness in the face of suffering and adversity; forbearance (a great word to know). A Word a Day even has a theme for each week; this week's is words from *The Devil's Dictionary* by Ambrose Bierce. You just open your e-mail and there it is. To subscribe, go to **www.wordsmith.org**.

Take Back the Key to Your Safety Deposit Box

Many of us feel that we can only be happy if other people say that we are worthwhile. We need others to tell us we did a good job or else we are afraid we haven't. We need others to say we are special, that we matter. Now, compliments are nice, indeed wonderful. But if we *must* have validation from others in order to feel good about ourselves, we are in what Dawna Markova calls a "spiritual emergency." It's as if we've given the key to the safety deposit box that holds our life savings to someone else. We can't access it ourselves; we have to go through them. What if they leave? What if they die, and we can't find the key? What if they steal the box? We can never experience true inner peace and contentment, because we're always wondering if the person with the key is going to disappear.

Ultimately what matters is that *you* feel good about who you are and what you are doing. And that is independent of praise, money, or material success—any other external factor. It's the quiet internal satisfaction that comes from knowing who you are and that you are contributing your best to the world.

Today, take a moment to remember that what matters is that you feel good about yourself.

Indulge in a Head Massage

Giving a head massage is easy and requires no formal training. All you need is someone who enjoys getting his or her head rubbed and is willing to reciprocate.

Stand behind the person and place your hands very gently on his or her head. Just rest there for a few seconds; the idea is to have the two of you relax together and for you to get in tune with him. If it is comfortable for him, have him close his eyes.

Place both hands on top of his head, so they meet at the midline. Using all the fingers of both hands, press and massage in circular motions, covering the entire scalp from forehead to nape of neck, and from ear to ear. Ask her to guide you as to how much pressure to apply. Use your thumbs on the spot where the base of the skull meets the neck.

Massage the temples in a firm, circular motion for a minute. Slowly massage your way across the forehead until your hands meet in the middle. Return to the temples and bring your hands down either side of her head to the point in front of the earlobes where the jaw tends to clench. Massage there. Finish off by gently pulling on his hair and tugging upward.

Find Your Simple
Pleasures of Summer

Today is the first day of summer. Hurrah! Maybe it's because of our experience with summer vacation as kids, but summer is the season that makes most of us the happiest. Eating outdoors, flowers bursting in yards, swimming, boating, water skiing, sailing, fresh cherries and nectarines. . . .

What are the little things that give you pleasure in the summer? Make a list and be sure to fit them all in this year.

Visualize Happiness

The actor Jim Carrey told *Women's World* magazine that when he was a kid, his family lost all their money and they had to live in a camper. To keep himself happy, he would "sit with my arms wide open and imagine I was holding a giant funnel with all good things pouring through it." By doing that, Jim created a self-fulfilling prophecy—he expected good things and thus noticed them when they came along.

You can do the same. Sit down and take a few deep, slow breaths. Now imagine yourself happy. Imagine that your relationships are better. Imagine your work is fulfilling. Imagine you feel good. See yourself as happy. Perhaps the image of a funnel works for you as well. If not, summon your own image of abundance. Allow yourself to receive the goodness from the universe.

Make Work Happier

I consider it an enormous privilege to do work that has meaning, work that is not only personally fulfilling but that also, I hope, can make a difference in the world. It's a privilege because many, if not most, people do not get such a sense of fulfillment from their jobs. Their work is something they do to put food on the table, something to endure in order to go home and do what really matters to them—play with their kids, wind surf, whatever.

But since we spend so much time at our jobs, no matter what we do, it's important to enjoy our time there as much as possible. Take a couple of minutes right now to think about how to make your work life more pleasurable. Is there any aspect of work that you like? Do you enjoy the people you work with? Can you bring some of what you do enjoy to the office—a former coworker loved to bake and would make all sorts of taste treats for us; another shares her progress in long-distance bike riding at staff meetings. Is there a benefit to society to what you do? What is it? Can you keep it in mind as you go about your day?

Today, find one thing about work that makes you happy.

Reach Out

Whenever you shut down connectedness, you get depressed.
—Glenda Taylor

The new physics teaches that we are all interconnected in ways that are elusive to our rational minds. We get glimpses of the truth of interconnection when we learn that people who are prayed for (without their knowing it) get better faster than others. Or when the same idea crops up suddenly in many different areas of the world without having been discussed or otherwise transferred. (I've become so convinced of this phenomenon that at Conari, we say that if we have an idea for a book we have to do it right that minute or another publisher will.)

Glenda Taylor reminds us that when we cut ourselves off (or more accurately, when we ignore, because I'm not sure we can be truly disconnected), we suffer. We get depressed because we feel alone, even though we're not really alone. It's an illusion, but a powerful one.

To keep our sense of connection alive, we need to continue to reach out. Even if we don't feel like it initially, the act of making contact will lighten our hearts. Join a chat room or support group, talk to someone new, volunteer one hour a week at a shelter. Staying connected keeps us uplifted.

Record a New Message on Your Answering Machine

I love it when I call two acquaintances, because they have such interesting messages on their answering machines. One recites her favorite poem of the moment; the other is exuberant about what she's doing and why she isn't there to take your call and finishes with: "You can leave offers to take me to dinner, or other delicious suggestions at the sound of the beep."

Spread some joy to your callers—tell a joke, offer an inspiring quotation, whatever will make you smile to record and them to hear.

Express a Bit More of Who You Are

So many of us end up in jobs or careers that do not reflect our true natures. Who are you really—a writer? An artist? A teacher? A public speaker? How can you bring a bit of that into your life? Take a painting class? Offer to teach a community college course? Volunteer at a hospice?

So many of us avoid the simple things that could reflect more of ourselves because we believe that we will be happy only if we make a big change—quit our job to become an artist, for example, rather than figuring out how to paint one hour a week. That all-or-nothing attitude keeps a lot of us from the satisfaction we could experience in our daily lives.

Today, think about one small thing you can do to express more of who you truly are. Remember the words of Joseph Campbell: "Hell is living someone else's life."

Bless the Day

Now when I awaken and before I even open my eyes, I thank the bed for a good night's sleep. After all, we have spent the whole night together in comfort. Then with my eyes still closed, I spend about ten minutes just being thankful for all the good in my life. I program my day a bit, affirming that everything will go well and that I will enjoy it all.

—Louise Hay

What if you were to start every day with such a beginning?

The Bread Solution

Do you crave carbohydrates? Whole grain breads and cereals are thought to aid in making us feel calm and happy because they help speed tryptophan, an amino acid, to the brain. Tryptophan increases the levels of serotonin, that magical chemical that makes us feel good.

That's why I'm convinced that every time I go on a diet, I turn into a snarling monster. While several diets extol the virtues of a high-protein, low-carbohydrate diet, most nutritionists believe that whole grains and cereals should make up a good portion of our daily meals.

So if you're feeling low, try a diet high in whole grain breads and cereals. Just avoid the high fat and sugar "go withs"—mayonnaise, cheese, jam—and you'll feel better without putting on pounds.

Haul Out the Photo Albums

The older the better. Look at yourself and friends and family in those funny clothes and haircuts. Remember that shack you used to live in? That old Beetle you used to drive? How cute your three-year-old daughter was in her tutu?

There's great fun in reminiscing, and photos are such a wonderful way to reconnect to the past. Take a trip through all your yesterdays.

Keep Happiness Momentos

I like to save the notes of thanks and appreciation that I have received over the years and when I need a little pick-me-up, I take them out and reread them. I remember again the person who sent the note, what the circumstances were—oh, that was the very nice intern who was so pleasant to be around—and bask in the glow of someone appreciating me.

You can do this with cards, e-mail, or voice mail. I have a friend who saves all the "love calls" she gets on her answering machine. Another friend writes down the compliments she receives in a journal and takes it out in time of need.

Being loved and appreciated is wonderful. Why not preserve those moments?

Go Wild, at Least a Little

Sometimes we just need to shake up our routine to feel better. What little outrageous thing can you do today? Dye your hair? Paint your toenails green? Play hooky from work?

For years, I lived near a street that must have had six or seven Chinese restaurants, and over time, I've probably eaten at them all. One day, I commented to my husband that each seemed to do a particular dish well and that if you put them all together, it would make a great meal. So one night, when we were feeling the need to be a bit outrageous, we did just that. We had potstickers from one place, then moved onto the next for hot and sour soup, a third for the Szechwan beef, and a fourth for the garlic eggplant. If anyone thought we were weird only ordering one item per restaurant, no one said anything. We had a ball—not to mention a great dinner.

Trade Love Lists

I had to learn this lesson the hard way. So much misery in relationships comes from our expecting that the other person, by virtue of loving us, should know exactly what makes us feel loved. But, as Daphne Rose Kingma says in her wise book *True Love,* your sweetheart isn't psychic and neither are you. Unless we are told, we tend to give what we want to receive, and that can lead to all kinds of frustration and resentment: Why does she always try to rub my back when I hate backrubs? Why does he send red roses when he should know I like pink?

To increase the happiness quotient in your relationship (any relationship), agree that the two of you will make a list of ten things that make you feel loved. Then trade lists and commit to doing one item on the list this week. (For advanced lovers, do one a week until you've run through the list. Make a new list or use this one again.)

Experience Sympathetic Joy

"I'm so happy for you." How often do you find yourself saying something like that? When we feel happiness for someone else, we are experiencing what Buddhists call "sympathetic joy," the true rejoicing in the good fortune of someone else. Sympathetic joy challenges some of our most closely-held assumptions, namely that happiness or success are finite qualities and that if someone else experiences them, somehow we will get less.

Sympathetic joy recognizes the interconnection between us—that my friend's happiness is in some sense truly my own. Indeed happiness actually grows as we share it because, as Sharon Salzberg notes, "The act of sharing puts us in touch with its source, which is limitless."

That being said, it isn't always easy to practice. Lots of things—envy, competition, bitterness—can stand in our way. A friend of mine just had a baby and when I went to see the two of them, rather than rejoicing with her wholeheartedly, I was filled with a sense of loss that I hadn't known my daughter until she was one year old. (She is adopted.) But as I became aware of what I was feeling, I could bow to that and hold her daughter tight, sending my cradling to my daughter's spirit.

Look around. Is someone in your life experiencing happiness? Can you rejoice with them?

Don't Wait

This has taken me a very long time to learn, and I can't say I do it all the time, but I am trying. In every single moment, we have the choice to be happy or not. No matter what is going on, we can choose to focus on what is right, what is good and whole in ourselves and our lives, and what options we have in any given situation. In other words, we can choose to be happy no matter what.

If we don't, then we get caught in the "as soon as" syndrome: As soon as my business is on a better footing, I'll be happy. As soon as my husband starts paying attention to me, I'll be happy. As soon as my back stops hurting, I'll be happy. This is a vicious trap I've spent decades in. But perhaps your back will not stop hurting. Perhaps your husband will never give you the kind of attention you desire. And if your "as soon as" comes to pass, chances are your happiness will be fleeting and another "as soon as" will crop up. That's because true contentment is not based on externals, but on an internal choice to turn, like a plant, toward the light.

Don't wait till your ship comes in to be happy. For it may never, and even if it does, you'll have missed out on the chance for joy between now and then. Say to yourself, "I choose to be happy today."

Lighten Up

Check out these two rib-tickling Web sites: **www.theonion.com** (a satirical weekly newspaper with articles like "North Dakota Not Heard from in 48 Hours"); **http://now2000.com/weird/** (a link to many hysterical sites including "Spam Haiku," all luncheon meat poetry, all the time).

Wake Up Naturally

Studies have shown that waking up to an alarm clock interrupts your body's natural circadian rhythms, which can negatively effect your mood for the rest of the day. So if you want to be happy, allow yourself to wake up on your own, when your body feels ready. If you must get up at a certain time, set a mental alarm. Tell yourself to wake up at 7 A.M., for example, and imagine a clock that says 7:00. Envision waking alert and ready for the day (experiment with setting a back-up clock). Researchers have found that most people will wake within a few minutes of the envisioned time, leading them to speculate that our biological clocks are in communication with our subconscious minds.

Do Nothing for a While

Tinker, putter, wander aimlessly. Just do something for the pure pleasure of it today. Read a book, weed the garden. . . . Whatever you choose, choose it because you want to do it, not because you have to or you should. How will you do nothing?

Make a Pick-Me-Up Drawer at Work

I can get so caught up in the minutiae of work that I forget what's important to me. That's why I have taken to looking at a picture of my daughter and husband on my desk when I get overstressed. It never fails to bring a smile to my face and brings me back to what's truly important. So when I read in a magazine about creating a drawer of happiness enhancers, I knew I had to try it at work. I shuffled my stuff around to empty out one whole desk drawer and have filled it with things that make me happy no matter what—photos, cards, dried roses, a carved stone that I love to touch. . . . It always lifts my spirit.

Give it a try.

Go Skinny Dipping

One of my great memories of childhood is of swimming naked at night in the lake by my house. The silky water on my skin, the kiss of the still-warm air, the stars twinkling. It is something I have never forgotten.

All you need is a little daring and access to a pool, lake, pond, ocean, or quarry. For added fun, convince someone to go with you, preferably a romantic partner.

Cool Down

When it's really hot, it's easy to feel miserable. As I write this, the thermometer is hovering at 100 degrees. Here's a quick skin refresher that you can splash on any time you're feeling hot and sticky. Bring 1 cup of water to a boil. Add ½ cup each finely grated lemon peel and grapefruit peel, and 1 cup of mint leaves. Boil for two minutes and then remove from heat. Cool and strain. Store in a glass bottle in the refrigerator for up to three weeks.

Take a Walk

Go to the reservoir or around the neighborhood. Walk downtown instead of driving. Feel your feet on the pavement and the sensation of your body moving at its own pace through time and space. Look for birds or squirrels; enjoy drinking in your surroundings with your eyes.

Because mind, body, spirit are interconnected, anything good for one is good for all aspects of yourself. In walking, your body gets exercised, your spirits are raised, and science has uncovered that even your mind is improved. According to a study conducted at the University of Illinois, formerly sedentary senior citizens had improved cognitive functioning after a six-month program of walking an hour three times a week. The mental benefits of walking were especially significant, researchers said, because the subjects had not exercised regularly previously. Interestingly, non-aerobic exercise such as stretching did not offer the same mental boost.

Overtip Today

I love this prescription for joy from Robert Fulghum. It not only brings a spot of pleasure into a hardworking person's life, but it expresses your faith in abundance, that you don't have to be stingy or withholding with your resources.

Fulghum's actual recommendation is to overtip a breakfast waitress, a woman who works long and hard for little compensation. It reminds me of a man I once knew who had a policy of tipping everyone the same amount. He argued that the waitress at a greasy spoon worked at least as hard as someone in the fanciest restaurant, and therefore a tip based on the percentage of the bill was not fair. He had worked out what he considered an average of all bills and tipped that no matter what. I think it was $10. The expression on the face of the person who just served him a $5 sandwich was priceless. (I was never with him when he offered the same to a waiter who had just served a $200 dinner.)

Whatever amount you choose, it's a wonderful way to life your spirits (and assure continued good service!).

Are You Responsible?

Those of us with training in pessimism tend to think we are responsible for things that go wrong, even if they are truly out of our control. Recently I felt terrible because I had planned an outdoor barbecue for out-of-town guests and the weather was cold so we had to eat indoors. I was miserable—I felt guilty about the poor *weather!* Talk about a situation out of my control!

The truth is we are accountable for certain things, and not others. If we renege on a promise, for example, it is appropriate to feel responsible. Knowing the difference goes a long way toward peace of mind. Is there something bothering you right now? Do you really have any accountability to it? Understanding what you are truly responsible for eliminates hopelessness and allows you to take appropriate action. And if you find yourself feeling responsible for everything on the face of the Earth, just notice that without judgment—oh, there I am again, feeling overly responsible. That way it's possible to let it go.

Discover Your Rosebush of Happiness

I took a different route to work the other day and came across something I had never seen before—a huge hedge full of vibrant pink roses as big as saucers. Immediately my spirit soared. I'd never seen a rose hedge! Now I drive that way every day, just so my eyes can drink in that beauty again.

As you go about your day, be alert to whatever might be in your surroundings that could give you such a boost. Is it the lovers holding hands as they walk down the street? The boy hugging his puppy? A field of poppies? Your rosebush of happiness awaits you.

Give Yourself Flowers—Just Because

This is an easy one, if you really do it. To get the most for your money, consider blooms that are particularly long lasting—sunflowers, Peruvian lilies, or dahlias are all good choices. But more important, go for what will bring a smile to your face.

What Is Your Heart Longing For?

This is a practice adapted from *Contentment* by Robert A. Johnson and Jerry M. Ruhl. Find a place to sit quietly for a few minutes. Take a few slow, deep breaths. Now think back over the past week. What have you spent your time, energy, and money doing? How has each thing contributed to your happiness or not? Now, continuing to breath calmly, turn your attention to your heart and ask, "What is my heart longing for?" Perhaps the answer will pop up immediately; perhaps it will surface later. If you do get an answer right away, compare it to your list of how you've been spending your time and money. Notice how you feel. Is there a way to invest more in what your heart is longing for?

Talk to a Friend

Happiness is in the comfortable companionship of friends.
—Pam Brown

When women in a survey were asked to define what made them glow—a sense of completely perfect happiness, even for a moment or two—the overwhelming response was talking to friends.

Today, call, write, or e-mail a beloved friend.

Trash Day

Here's an antidote to chronic worry. Write down every problem you have on a piece of paper, one piece for each problem. Make a stack. Read the top paper in the stack. Spend a few minutes thinking about how to solve the problem and then throw the paper in the trash can. Repeat until the whole stack is gone. Then tell yourself you won't think about your worries again till tomorrow. That's it.

This technique works on the theory that most chronic worry is just an endless feedback loop—your mind spins around and around about the same things over and over. Here you allow yourself to think about each problem, but not obsess about it. This allows you to focus on finding solutions, and not just spin. It also allows you peace of mind for the rest of the day—you've done your worry work and can now relax.

Offer an Adjective

I think it is a truism that no one can receive too much genuine praise. It is such a great morale and ego booster. It helps us feel seen, to keep going, to feel good about ourselves. Children, mates, coworkers—everyone needs as much praise as possible, including ourselves!

Recently a coworker suggested a practice of praise that was incredibly easy. Here's how you do it in a work setting. Write down on small pieces of paper one positive adjective to describe each person you work with (so if you have ten colleagues you have ten pieces of paper and ten different adjectives). Then you deliver the papers anonymously. We put them in staff mailboxes. Then later, everyone collected all their adjectives. I was flabbergasted to see how others saw me. People said such praising things that they would never say to my face. I took all the papers and made a collage that I still pull out and look at when I'm feeling blue.

You can adapt this in any way you want. In a family, you could do five adjectives each, perhaps. It also makes a great birthday or anniversary card.

Sing in the Shower or Your Car

Many people die with their music still in them.
—Oliver Wendell Holmes

When I was a kid, I loved to sing. I sang in the choir and was often chosen to do solos (because of the loudness of my voice, not its quality). But as I got older, I got embarrassed about my voice and stopped singing.

Sound familiar? So many of us have cut ourselves off from this natural joy maker. It's too bad because singing lifts our spirits and opens our hearts. And it's been shown to lower blood pressure and alleviate depression and sleep disorders.

So sing today, even one short silly song. If you find singing in public too intimidating, wait until you are your only audience.

What Stands Out?

Make a list of the five most memorable experiences of your life. What made each memorable? Does it offer any clues as to what brings you the most joy?

Now, if it feels right, consider sharing your list with someone close to you.

Open Your Pores

Open all your pores and bathe in all the tides of nature.
—Henry David Thoreau

Summer is such a wonderful time to revel in nature—the grass between your bare toes, the tickle of saltwater as it dries on your skin, the smell of rain on hot asphalt. When I was a kid, one of my favorite things to do was to run outside in a warm rain. I especially loved to stand under the drain spout and let the water cascade on my head.

Today, take Thoreau's advice and bathe in nature.

How Much Is Enough?

This question is posed by environmentalist Bill McKibben. It is one of the most significant questions of our time, for depending how we answer, our very life—and the life of all other beings on this planet—may be jeopardized.

But it is also a significant question for cultivating happiness because it's so easy, particularly in this consumer culture, to think happiness will come from more stuff—more clothes, a bigger house, a fancier car, another computer. The truth of course is that material objects can bring us pleasure, but not the deep lasting contentment that a rich inner life, loving relationships, and meaningful work can. It's a vicious cycle—the more we run after possessions, the more we can lose focus of what truly matters, and the more in debt we get, forcing us to focus even more intently on money.

How much is enough for you?

Look Inside Yourself

According to the Rutgers University National Marriage Project, Americans are less likely than ever to be "very happy" in their marriages. The percentage of people who reported being very happy fell from 53.5 percent in the 1970s to 37.8 percent in 1996. The study did not purport to analyze why, but one of my guesses is the fact that we tend to have unrealistic expectations for our relationships, expecting the other person to make all our dreams come true.

Yup. Happiness is each and every one of our personal responsibilities. A mate can augment our happiness, give us something to be happy about, but he or she can't *make* us happy.

Are you looking outside yourself for satisfaction?

Ask and Ye Shall Receive

What would you like to receive today to bring you a spot of happiness? Imagine it for a minute, then surround it in your mind with a pink bubble of love and imagine the bubble ascending into space. Then open yourself to receiving your request—but remember it may not come in the exact way, shape, form, or timing that you expected.

Getting an Eyeful

In her very useful book *The Pleasure Zone,* therapist Stella Resnick offers a number of personal experiments for increasing pleasure. One that I love helps us to increase pleasure through our eyes. Here's how:

"In a relaxed and experimental frame of mind, look around the area surrounding you and see what pleases you visually. You may see a print in a frame or a pretty view out your window. Look for vividness of color, a pattern of geometric shapes, lines converging and separating, a metallic sheen or patina, a play of light and shadows. . . .

"Then close your eyes and see what you can recall of what you just saw. What images or colors stand out for you? Open your eyes and compare the true image with what you imagine." Enhancing visual memory sharpens our ability to truly see what is in front of us, the world in all its majesty and splendor.

Walk in Dewy Grass

I love this suggestion. I found it in *Chicken Soup and Other Folk Remedies* by Joan Wilen and Lydia Wilen. It is a remedy for fatigue, but I find it to be one of the swiftest happiness enhancers I know. Maybe because I love going barefoot so much, and the added bonus of wet grass is simply delicious.

If your access to dewy grass is limited, the Wilens suggest an alternative—"Next best thing is to carefully walk up and back in 6 inches of cold bathwater. Do it for 5 to 10 minutes in the morning and late afternoon."

Keep a Sense of Proportion

"How are you today, Mom?"

"I'm fine—if you overlook a few things."

— A conversation between author David Kundtz
and his mother

What wise advice! As David Kundtz points out in his new book *Everyday Serenity,* each of us is presented daily with all kinds of "opportunities to overlook a few things: my own aches and pains, failings, frustrations, moments of impatience; or another person's fumbling, forgetfulness, or other foibles." Any time something goes wrong, we can choose to be annoyed, impatient, angry, or we can shrug our shoulders and think to ourselves, "No big deal."

Some of the most unhappy people I know have the most trouble with this. Everything is a major crisis, every mistake is the end of the world. Lacking a sense of proportion, they drive themselves and those around them crazy.

Do yourself a favor. Overlook at least two things today.

Have Some Real Fun

I recently read a manuscript that claimed that more people spend time in casinos than any other recreational venue. And that people lost $50.9 billion in gambling in 1997, which exceeded the amount spent on movies, sports, theme parks, and CD purchases *combined*.

I don't know what that means to you, but to me it seems like a lot of people have lost touch with real fun, true play. True play involves us creatively, fosters spontaneity, even silliness, fills us with joy, and connects us beyond words to our playmates. In a phrase, it makes us more alive. Play isn't supposed to enslave us, bankrupt us, or disconnect us from one another.

Almost all of us have had our natural playfulness erode as we've grown up, and we may find it downright difficult to have real fun. If that's true for you, I suggest borrowing a preschooler, but you can also go it alone. Jump on your spouse lying on the bed. Or have a tickle fight. Or go on a walk where each of you takes turns calling out a direction when you come to an intersection. Get down on the floor and play with blocks.

Really Taste Your Food

Part of what takes us away from joy in our lives is that our senses become numb. We lose the natural exuberance of early childhood, when everything was miraculous. But we can reawaken our senses to the sheer wonder of being alive. One great way is with what is called the "Eating Meditation."

All you need is a few—two or three—raisins or chocolate kisses. (Actually any small piece of food that you like will do, but I'm going to instruct you as if it were a raisin.) Sit down and place one raisin in front of you. Really look at it. Notice its shape, color, texture. Think of all the work that went into getting it from bare earth to your table. Now, very slowly, pick it up and smell it. What does it smell like? What does it remind you of? Now, again moving very slowly, place it in your mouth. Roll it around a bit on your tongue and see what flavors you can taste without chewing. Just let it sit there a while. Finally, when you can't wait any longer, bite down and chew very slowly, experiencing all you can from the taste. Really savor it. Now swallow. Repeat with another raisin if desired.

I'm not going to tell you what you will experience, because everyone has their own response to this. But I can say that it will be the best raisin you ever had in your life.

Feel Peppier

If you've been dragging around, it's hard to feel happy. You might want to try a new coenzyme supplement that researchers have recently become interested in: Enada NADH. NADH is found naturally in beef, fish, chicken, and turkey, but our bodies can process only a small amount from food. In studies, 31 percent of those who took NADH supplements felt perkier in two weeks and 71 percent ultimately felt more energetic. You can purchase this and other health supplements online—see the entry for March 5 for the Web sites.

Learn from Those around You

Often the people in our lives are our greatest teachers. Some folks say that we attract precisely the people we need in our lives to learn what we have to learn.

We learn from them not only directly—oh, so that's how to do it—but also by negative example—oh, so that's how *not* to do it. We learn from them by having to stretch ourselves in new ways—to assert ourselves finally, maybe, to avoid being run over by someone. Or to be more patient and tolerant of mistakes. When we see our interactions as opportunities for growth, we can be happier with them and with ourselves.

The list of what we might be learning is endless and different for each one of us. But today, I'd like you to contemplate these two questions: From whom must I learn to receive? From whom (or what) must I learn to protect myself? Take note of your answers and stay open.

Look for the Happiness under Your Nose

While you're on you way to your pot of gold,
don't forget to pick up the silver along the way.
—Anonymous

How often do we ignore the silver in our path because we're so focused on that pot of gold? I do it all the time. I aim for a goal, and then spend all my mental energy trying to make it happen and being upset that it hasn't happened yet, oblivious to the good things that are right under my nose.

Right now, think of five pieces of silver in your life you've failed to notice and appreciate. Here's my list: my good health, the health of my family, my resiliency and resourcefulness, my love of learning, my comfortable house.

Go on a Complaint Fast

When asking people about happiness for this book, one friend turned to another and said, "What *do* we do to be happy? It seems like we spend most of our time grousing and complaining." Boy, did I recognize myself in that remark.

It was medical intuitive Caroline Myss who popularized the notion that we Americans bond over our pain, our victimhood. We love to talk to one another about all the ways and whys of our woundings. But as she points out, that keeps us stuck in our pain, unable to move on.

Have you been playing your violin a bit too often, singing the old song of how terribly the world treats you? Or perhaps you've just focused on the terrible traffic, the lousy weather, the inconsiderateness of bank tellers.

Whatever your favorite litany of complaints is, commit to a twenty-four-hour moratorium on complaining. First notice how often you tend to do it. Then be aware of what you mind does instead.

Chill Out

When it's hotter than hell, take a happiness tip from the character Marilyn Monroe played in *The Seven Year Itch*. Chill your underwear in the refrigerator before getting dressed.

What's Easier These Days?

No matter what your life circumstances, no matter what you are going through right now, because of the work you've done on yourself, some things are easier, if only because your ability to roll with the punches has improved.

Take a few moments right now to look at your life as a whole and reflect on what has become easier. Your intimate relationships? Your parenting? Your effectiveness in dealing with a difficult person? Your ability to give up perfectionism? Whatever it is, take a minute to celebrate those things, and allow them to remind you that life *can* improve.

Re-live Happy Moments

Sometimes the best thing we can do for ourselves when we face a task is to relive the excitement, joy, and good feelings we experienced when we did something similar before. That will put us into a positive frame of mind to tackle the new task.

For example, writing a book can be hard. But when I remember how good it feels to get letters from readers whose lives have changed for the better as a consequence of what I've written, I get an upsurge of energy that carries me along.

Giving a speech? Recall the last time when people flooded the podium afterward to say thanks. Doing a report? Remember the praise your team got for the great idea you generated last year. Tap into those positive feelings and ride on the energy they generate.

Take a Cool Shower

The benefits of water have long been known for treating injuries. But recently there has been growing interest in the benefits of hydrotherapy to prevent sickness and reduce stress. And medicine is now discovering what we intuitively have known all along—that the temperature of the water produces different effects: warm water is relaxing and puts you to sleep; cold water invigorates. Much attention is now being paid to contrast showers where you alternate hot and cold, which are said by some holistic healers to be the fastest way to achieve good health.

Because it's August, I'm going to suggest you try an energy-boosting cool shower from *The Complete Book of Water Healing.* It will elevate your mood and combat fatigue by making your blood circulate faster. Stand under warm water for two to three minutes, then gradually make the water cooler and cooler, standing under cold water for two minutes.

Go Out on a Date with Yourself

What do you love to do that you haven't done in a long time? Ride horseback? Swim in the ocean? See a double feature? Get a massage? Make a date with yourself to do it.

Log On to Heartwarmers

Heartwarmers4u.com is a free e-mail service that sends a new inspirational story six days a week (never on Sunday!). Most of the material is original and comes from members who send in their own stories of hope, courage, and humor. They also recommend other inspirational Internet sites, such as A Ray of Sunshine Rhymes (**www.rytebyte.com/rhymeworld/array/**) and Funny Kids (**www.funnykids.com**). To join, e-mail **heartwarmers-on@heartwarmers4u.com**. Guaranteed to make you feel good!

Build a Sandcastle

What fun! All you need is a few large and small buckets, shovels and trowels, and spoons. You'll attract plenty of young helpers. Pick a flat spot where the tide is going out. And don't forget the sunscreen!

If you want to go high tech, check out **www.sandsculpture.com**, where professional sand sculptors share their secrets.

The Grand Adventure

What if you decided today that whatever was going on in your life was a grand adventure? How would that change your day?

Just yesterday, my car died on the way to work (only weeks after spending too much on engine repairs), and then a full cup of coffee shattered as I was fumbling with the front office keys. Instead of giving in to anger and frustration, I stepped back and saw my morning as an "Aren't Mondays Horrible?" drama. Viewing it from a distance, it started to look much more comic than tragic, and I felt much better.

Create Some Luck

Have you ever said, "If it weren't for my bad luck, I'd have no luck at all"? Does it seem like only other people enjoy good luck? According to Marc Myers, author of *How to Make Luck,* luck is not random at all. It's just that certain people are better at making good luck than others. Here's how to do it, he claims:

1. Instead of envying other people's luck, make a list of what is positive in your life. Envy saps luck-attracting energy.

2. Really connect when you meet people—smile warmly, look in their eyes, remember their name. A chance meeting often brings luck.

3. Let go of mistakes quickly by focusing on the positive.

4. Write down your goals and the people who can help you make them happen.

5. Make time and space for opportunity to knock. If you're too busy running around distracted, you won't recognize a lucky break when it occurs.

Give Up Grudges

A grudge is a contraction of the heart, a holding back from positive feelings. When we hold a grudge, it stands in the way of love and happiness flowing in and out of our lives.

There's a wonderful Zen teaching story about that. Two monks were traveling on foot and came across a stream. A woman who had injured her ankle trying to cross was sitting by the stream. Even though it is taboo for monks to touch women, one of the monks, seeing her dilemma, carried her on his back to her village a short way away. Then the two monks went on in silence for many hours. Finally, the other monk spoke, criticizing the first monk for breaking his vow by touching the woman. The compassionate monk turned to his companion, saying quietly, "I put her down miles ago. You're still carrying her."

What old grudge are you still carrying that you can put down? Do it now in the quiet of your own heart.

Lavish Yourself with Attention

What would happen if you lavished attention on yourself? What would happen if you treated yourself with the same kind of attention you give your spouse, your children, your friends? How would you behave differently?

Calm Down with Passionflower

Passionflower has been used for centuries to relieve stress and anxiety, and to promote sound sleep. It can be found in many forms—pills, capsules, powders—in health food stores, but herbalists claim that it is most effective taken as a tea. A good starting dose is one or two cups of tea before bedtime. It's been proven to be safe in moderate doses, but should not be taken in large amounts because it can lead to over-sedation, especially when mixed with prescription drugs or other herbs. To be safe, consult your doctor before taking this or any other herb.

Don't Compare

One of the quickest ways to get miserable is to compare your life with that of someone you perceive to have it better than you. First, you can't really compare because you can never know what their life is like on the inside. Second, it is totally irrelevant to who you are and what you are supposed to be doing with *your* life.

I was reminded of this recently in a delightful way by Iyanla Vanzant. She was writing about sitting in her expensive Jacuzzi, reveling in her newfound prosperity, when she noticed that her dog had messed all over the carpet. "Life is about cleaning up the crap and, while you're doing it, being OK with the fact that you have to do it," she philosophized. "You can't get caught up in the right or wrong, good or bad, injustice or unfairness of cleaning up the crap in your life. You cannot compare how much of it you have to the amount someone else may have." You just have to clean it up happily.

We all have our share of crap to clean. The trick is to do it with a willing heart.

What's the Worst Thing That Could Happen?

To see and know the worst is to take from Fear her main advantage.
—Charlotte Brontë

As Bronte so brilliantly points out, sometimes the best way to handle our fears is to play them out all the way. That way they lose some of their power because we have mentally faced the worst and survived. It's also a good way to remember that everything that happens, no matter how difficult, can be used as spiritual grist for the mill.

Here's how to do it. Pick one of your fears. Then play it out by asking yourself, "And then what happens?" after each thought. For example, one of my fears is going bankrupt. So I ask myself, "And then what happens?"

"Then I lose my house with the swimming pool and all my savings." "And then what happens?" "I have to live in an apartment and take a job that has a retirement plan." "And then what happens?" "I guess I'd become a teacher because it has a retirement program and I am qualified." "And then what happens?" "I would probably enjoy it."

Now you might be thinking, "But my fear won't end up so rosy," but you'd be surprised. This technique helps you engage your resourcefulness, to figure out what you would do in a difficult circumstance. It's a very powerful booster.

Just Do Something

The state of the world, the country, the community, the neighborhood can really get you down. And it's easy to slip into despair, believing that one person can't make a difference, so why even try. But the world is full of stories of people who decided to take action and ended up having a huge impact—for instance, the woman who started Mothers Against Drunk Drivers (MADD) after her daughter was killed by a drunk driver. With MADD's help, drunk driving has declined every year since the group's inception. Or four-year-old Isis Johnson, who asked her grandmother one day, "Can we send the chicken we have left to the children in Ethiopia?" From that question she and her grandmother founded the Isis Johnson Foundation, which collects food and clothing for needy Louisianians.

If you have no time, do something small—write a letter to the editor of your local paper about a local problem that's bugging you. Or consider joining 20/20 Vision, an organization that tracks national and international events and sends a suggested "action" each month they say will take only twenty minutes at the most—often it's a call or a letter to a politician. To learn more about them call 202-833-2020, or e-mail **vision@2020vision.org**.

Try Walking Meditation

Now before I explain this, I want to say, "To each his or her own." I happen to dislike walking meditation, but other people swear by it. So see if it works for you. The idea is to slow your walking way down, so that you can be conscious of the process, rather than just doing it without thinking.

Set a timer for ten minutes to start. Find a spot indoors or out that is at least ten to twenty feet long. (You might want to do this where no one can see you, if you might feel self-conscious.) Stand still and notice that you are standing still. Feel your body standing, then feel the pressure of the earth on the soles of your feet. Now, very slowly, lift one leg, noticing that you are lifting your leg and reach out to take a step. As you place your foot, notice that you are placing your foot. Then notice your weight shifting in preparation to lift the other foot. Repeat. Keep going until you reach the end of your space, then turn around and walk slowly back to where you started.

As you slowly walk, your mind will wander off. When you notice it has, bring it back to the act of walking—lifting, placing, lifting, placing. Note your urge to see how much time is left. As Sylvia Boorstein says in *Don't Just Do Something, Sit There,* "Just walk. Remember, there's nowhere to go. You're already there."

Get (or Give) a Pep Talk

I can't tell you how many times I get cheered up in the act of cheering someone else up. I first noticed this in college with my boyfriend Rick. I would be moping around, and then he'd sink down. Because I couldn't stand *both* of us being depressed, I would launch into a speech about all the things still worth living for. Soon both of us were laughing.

If you're so down that you can't get up yourself, call someone you know and ask for a boost. Be specific—say something like, "Remind me why I should be happy."

Open to a Little Miracle

A little miracle is a burst of unexpected happiness. It comes out of the blue to delight us with its complete unanticipatedness. Rainbows are little miracles. So is a catch-up call from someone you haven't heard from in years. My coworker Suzanne told me of one she experienced last weekend: "I rode my bike up to the top of the mountain and there, in the field in front of me, were thousands of dragonflies!"

Today, watch for a little miracle. You just never know where it might be.

What Do You Need to Let Go Of?

Often we are most unhappy when we are stuck in some outdated mode of being and afraid to let go because we are invested in that old image of ourselves. We are stuck in a job we hate because we're convinced we need the house with the swimming pool. Or the status the job brings socially. Or the image of ourselves as powerful in a particular field. Or we drift along in an unsatisfying marriage because we are afraid to not be in a relationship. We cling to the status quo because the familiar is comfortable.

When we do, however, we forget that we are just as much a part of nature as everything else in the world. And nature has cycles—things are born, blossom, wilt, and die. So do aspects of ourselves. At any given moment, old ways of being may be dying and new ones aching to be born. We interrupt and delay this natural cycle, and cause ourselves to suffer from stagnation, when we cling to something past its time.

Right now, what do you need to let go of? A job that you have outgrown? A habit of relating to others? Negative thinking? Leaving the familiar is scary, but it is also exciting. For now, just notice what you are clinging to that needs to be let go of. As you do, you will signal to yourself that you are ready to embrace the new.

Try the Herbal Prozac

If you suffer from mild depression, you might benefit from St. John's Wort, a medicinal herb that has garnered much attention in the past few years. In fact, the herb has been used for over 2,000 years as a stress, anxiety, and insomnia remedy, and it has been well researched in Europe. Indeed, research shows that it is as effective as prescription antidepressants, but with fewer side effects (although there haven't been many studies on the effects of taking it long term). Over 20 million Germans currently take St. John's Wort for depression.

The trick is the dosage. Effective doses vary from person to person and, like prescription antidepressants, it can take several weeks to kick in. Herbalists recommend starting with 300 mg containing 0.3 percent hypercin (the active ingredient). (The best-researched formula is called Kira.) Through trial and error, you should be able to see what dose, taken at what time of the day, works for you. Many people take 100 mg at each meal. Side effects include increased sensitivity to sun, irritability, allergic reactions, and tiredness. Don't try it without talking to your doctor, particularly if you are on prescription antidepressants.

Blow Bubbles

This requires a bit of money—89 cents or so. Go out and buy an eight-ounce bottle of bubbles, find a small child or receptive adult, a good spot outside, and let yourself go. I guarantee you'll have a good time. Watch how the wind carries them hither and yon. Blow a few on the other person and see if they can catch them. Allow yourself the indulgence of being two years old again, if only for fifteen minutes.

Do Music Therapy

I don't sing because I'm happy. I'm happy because I sing.
—William James

As a teen and young adult, I loved to wallow in misery. I would put on sad music and really allow myself to sink down. My husband would always know as soon as he walked in the door. He'd see me in a puddle on the floor and say, "You've been listening to Leonard Cohen again, haven't you?" Eventually I grew out of it.

Music is a very powerful mood elevator and suppressor. To be happy, listen to music that makes you feel good, whether that's through inspiring lyrics or the rhythm of the piece. Make a tape or CD with ten or twelve songs that are your favorite uppers. Play it when you want a little lift.

Dance on Paper

This is a practice from *The Well-Being Journal* by Lucia Capaccione.

"Play some music that expresses your mood. If you want to feel more upbeat, play something that gets you snapping your fingers. With your nondominant hand, scribble or doodle to the music. Don't try to draw a picture or representational image. Just let your pen, pencil, or crayon move freely on the paper as though you were dancing. Your drawing will be like the tracks skaters leave on the ice. As you draw be aware of the movement of your arms and shoulders. Let the rhythm fill your entire body."

The Four Winds of Feelings

At every given moment, says my friend Daphne Rose Kingma, we have a jetstream of feelings operating below our conscious awareness. By bringing these feelings into consciousness, we begin to acquaint ourselves more fully with our deeper selves, and increase our capacity for joy by experiencing the full range of our feelings. For if we cut ourselves off from any feeling, we cut ourselves off from the capacity to feel all the others as well. To truly know our joy, we must also know our anger, our sadness. It's an all-or-nothing arrangement.

Because so many of us are cut off from our feelings (or at least some of our feelings), she advocates what she calls "the four winds of feelings." It requires answering four questions: What am I happy about? What am I sad about? What am I angry about? What am I afraid of? Try it and see if you can connect with the full richness of your feelings.

Become a Vehicle for Divine Energy

Julia Cameron, author of the bestselling *The Artist's Way*, has also written a beautiful little book entitled *Blessings*. It contains a meditation I find powerful for connecting to our hearts, one sure-fire way to experience joy. May it bring you happiness:

"My heart is a chalice for love. I am well loved. I open my heart to feel that I am loved. I allow myself to be saturated by love. I soften my heart and gently ask it to receive the love I encounter. I do not need to earn love. I do not need to work at love. I need only to allow myself to feel the love extended toward me. I need only to accept love to know that I am lovable. I choose to remember—and cherish—the ways in which I am loved."

Recognize this Truth

In his important book *The Road Less Traveled,* M. Scott Peck said something that changed my life: "Life is difficult. This is a great truth, one of the greatest truths. It is a great truth because once we truly see this truth, we transcend it. . . . Because once it is accepted, the fact that life is difficult no longer matters."

Where did we get the idea that life should be easy? That it should be effortless if we are doing the "right" thing? When my husband gets down, he often bemoans, "But life is so hard." Yes, I respond, it is. But, as Scott Peck says, the more we can accept life's difficulties, the more we can be happy despite the hardship. Because we've stopped resisting the challenges and accepted them as natural. It's not anything we're doing wrong, we're not bad or spiritually unevolved or undeserving—it's just that each life has a measure of difficulty.

Do you hold the belief that if you were doing "it" right, life would be easy? It's a tremendous happiness inhibitor.

Diversify

Everyone knows that in the stock market, diversification creates safety—put all your savings in one stock and you are very vulnerable if anything happens to that company. Spread your money around, and you'll also be spreading the risk and the potential to make substantial money.

The same is true for happiness. We need to cultivate a number of things that will make us happy, so we have a diverse portfolio on which to rely.

I didn't figure this out till my thirties. The only thing I knew how to do that I loved was reading. Now that's fine, but it's pretty limited. One day a friend said that I had to learn how to do something else and taught me needlepoint. I really enjoyed it and went on a needlepointing frenzy. Everyone I knew got pillows and eyeglass cases as gifts for years.

Then I developed repetitive stress disorder and had to give up needlepoint. Fortunately, I had diversified my happiness options in the meantime, so it was not an irreplaceable loss: I turned to cooking, swimming, writing, and more.

What new activity can you fold into your happiness portfolio?

Is Diet the Culprit?

If you find yourself suffering from a great deal of anxiety for no apparent reason, it might be caused by what you're eating. The main culprit is caffeine. According to research at the National Institute of Mental Health, drinking four cups of coffee a day can elevate your stress hormones and blood pressure by as much as 32 percent. They claim that women with full-blown anxiety have cured themselves without drugs simply by eliminating caffeine. If you want to try this, don't forget that caffeine is present not only in coffee but in tea, many kinds of soda, and chocolate.

The other culprit is sugar. For some people, sugary foods can cause extreme blood sugar fluctuations, which cause the adrenal glands to produce stress hormones. Instead of a donut, a cookie, or a piece of cake for a snack, reach for fruit, vegetables, or whole grain crackers. A side benefit is that you will up your intake of vitamins B and C, both known to help reduce anxiety.

Create a Mission Statement

In recent years, companies have created mission statements to create alignment among employees, to create a sense of higher purpose for the company's activities, and to articulate to customers the reason for the companiy's existence. Today, I am suggesting that you give some thought to creating your own personal mission statement.

Often we are unhappy because we get caught up in the swirl of daily life and have no sense of why we're doing what we're doing. We're on a treadmill, going 'round and 'round, having lost any sense of where we're going. That's why creating a mission statement is so powerful. It is an articulation of what you are doing and helps you see beyond the grind to the deeper purpose of your life. It can help you make changes when you see that your life is not in alignment with your deeper purpose.

Here's an example: My mission is to live my values as much as possible, so there is no discrepancy between my espoused beliefs and my behavior.

Take a few minutes right now to articulate your mission. Then paste it where you can see it.

Change for the Good

Just reading about this great new program makes me smile. Whenever I've traveled out of the country, I have felt bad when I return home with a few pesos or lire; once I even tried to convert them at my bank. They laughed at me! Fortunately, a great organization, Change for the Good, realized that a tremendous amount of money is wasted—$72 million a year to be exact—when low denomination money isn't exchanged. So they devised a system of collecting such funds to help needy kids worldwide. No amount is too small—only $2 can purchase 25 oral rehydration packets for starving kids. Since 1991, they've collected over $19 million in money most of us would have just thrown away.

If you fly on American, British Airways, or Air France, there is an envelope you can put your foreign coins in. If not, you can just mail bills and coins to Change for the Good, c/o Unicef, 333 E. 38th St., 6th Floor, New York, NY 10016.

Honor Your Contribution

Right around this time of year, we celebrate Labor Day. The holiday honors the workforce. In honor of that, take a few minutes right now to think about the work you do. Everyone works, whether at home, an office, or school. Think about what you contribute to your household, your community, and the world through the work you do. Give thanks to yourself for the labor you contribute.

Cherish

The other day I was doing a radio interview for my book, *Attitudes of Gratitude,* and the interviewer said that she thought one of the big problems with the world today is that we've forgotten how to cherish.

I don't think I've ever used or heard anyone else use the word. The dictionary tells us the primary meaning is "to hold dear; to treat with tenderness." In this disposable, use-it-up-and-throw-it-out, get-bored-quickly society, do we hold dear enough? Do we hold our loved ones dear? Do we cherish our possessions—the sturdy old car that still works for us, the sweater we've had for twenty years?

There is a kind of quiet contentment that comes from truly cherishing what we have. Look around you right now. What things in your life can you cherish?

Go Easy Today

There is a Buddhist proverb that goes, "Do without doing and everything gets done." I've certainly found it to be true. The more I approach something with a sense of ease, the easier it turns out to be.

How will you bring that sense of ease into your day today?

Share the Chores Equally

Study after study shows that working women do more than their fair share of the housework; the most recent study of 1,200 men and women by a researcher at Brown University found that women did 70 percent!

That same study, however, did something no other had done—it correlated happiness with the amount of work done and found, not surprisingly, that the bigger the woman's share, the more likely she was to feel depressed. And even more fascinating was that the amount of time a woman spent on housework wasn't significant; what mattered to her happiness was that the work, however long it took, be equally divided. Women who were happiest did no more than 46 percent (these spouses did about the same and kids and hired help took up the slack).

Are the chores divvied up fairly equally in your home?

Create a Pleasure/Pain List

This idea is inspired by Jonathan Robinson in *Shortcuts to Bliss*. On a piece of paper, make two vertical columns. In column one, write down ten things you like to do. In column two, write down ten things you hate to do. Then estimate the number of hours per month you spend doing each and add up the totals for each column.

Jonathan tells the story of a depressed client, James, who did this exercise. No wonder he was depressed and in constant conflict with his wife, says Jonathan. James spent 215 hours per month on things that he hated and only thirty-two hours per month on things he loved.

How's your ratio? If you're spending too little time doing things you love, chances are you aren't as happy as you could be. Is there a way to increase the "pleasure" column and decrease the "pain"?

Realize You Can't Have It All

A big block to happiness is thinking we can have everything we desire. When we fail to achieve that impossible goal, we are miserable. The truth is that *everything* is a trade-off. For example, if we work all the time to create material success, we may miss chances to be with our children as they grow, to be together at dinnertime, to develop other aspects of ourselves.

Happiness requires hard choices. To find it, we must be very clear on what is most important to us, and then arrange our lives so that we put those things first. If having a big fancy house will make you happy, great. If having meaningful work, even if it pays less, is most important, that's it. You are the only one who can be the judge of what will truly make you happy.

Right now, sit quietly and make a list of your top three priorities for happiness.

Receive with Joy

Whatever I am offered in devotion with a pure heart—
a leaf, a flower, fruit, or water—I accept with joy.
—Krishna

SEPTEMBER
9

We are continually being given to—by our friends, our family members, coworkers, life itself—and we can easily be blind to the gifts. As you go about your day, notice just *one* thing you are being given today, and receive it with joy.

Where Are You Right Now?

It's so easy to get caught up in the mundanities of life and lose track of the big picture of our lives. To keep focused on what is most significant, Dawna Markova has taken to orienting herself by asking four questions that she's shared with me: "What are you moving away from? What are you moving against? What are you moving with? What are you moving toward?"

Don't worry if you aren't sure what the questions mean. Just respond with the first thing that pops into your head. It's a powerful practice for getting clear on where you are right now in your life.

Feel Your Love

Here's a great happiness creator. Think of someone you love. Ask yourself, "What is it about that person that's so lovable?" As you think of the person's positive traits, allow yourself to feel your love and appreciation for them. See if you can feel your heart open. Do this practice any time today when you feel angry, fearful, or depressed, and let the loving sensations comfort you.

SEPTEMBER

11

Send an Animated Card

This is a pleasure of the e-mail age: sending animated cards to other e-mailers. There are all kinds of sites that offer these now, and many are free; **www.cardcentral** is a listing of free greeting card sites on the Internet. You can also look on

SEPTEMBER

12

www.gogreet.com

www.bluemountain.com

www.postcards.org/postcards

www.comedycentral.com/greetings

www.marlo.com.

Get a New Haircut

This is a tried and true pick-me-up. When feeling down, change the style or color of your hair. It really works—particularly if you end up with a great new look. I recently changed my hairstyle after having it the same for a few years, and everyone I met in the next few months told me how great I looked.

I should have done it sooner!

Help Someone Today

There is a wonderful, mystical law of nature that the three things we crave most in life—happiness, freedom, and peace of mind—are always attained by giving them to someone else.

—Anonymous

Helping others makes us feel good about ourselves. In case you need scientific confirmation, there is plenty. To cite just one: A recent study at Cornell University found that volunteering increasing a person's energy, sense of mastery over life (a measure of happiness), and self-esteem.

So why not give it a try? It can be as little as one hour a week. The world needs the gifts that only you have to offer.

Make a New Friend

So many of us despair that we have no time for the friends we have, so how can we fold another person into our lives? But new friends can add zest and excitement into our lives by offering different outlooks, activities, and experiences. And study after study has shown that the more friends you have, the healthier you'll be.

The latest in this research even shows that the more friends you have, the better you'll be protected from stress-related illnesses. In a study at Penn State University, researcher Mark Roy found that people's blood pressure rises (setting the stage for heart disease) when faced with stressors such as divorce, moving, or job loss. But the more friends a subject had (in this case firefighters), the faster their blood pressure would decrease, protecting them from the possible damaging effects of a long-term rise. The fewer friends a man had, the longer his blood pressure stayed elevated when faced with a difficult situation.

So keep yourself open to the possibility of increasing your friendship network. You'll be doing your heart a big favor.

Know the Magic Formula

In his book *Happiness Is Serious Business,* Dennis Prager points out a surefire formula for misery: U = I - R, which stands for Unhappiness equals Image minus Reality. What he means is that the more we have a set idea or image of how something will be, the more we will be disappointed by the reality of what is. We have an image of the way a relationship should be, and ours doesn't measure up. We have an image of what our lives are supposed to be like by the time we are forty, and we fall short. The more we create an image, the more we get in our own way of appreciating what is and the more we set ourselves up for unhappiness.

Does this sound familiar? If this is a trap you fall into, the best way out is to begin to recognize it: Oh, I thought it was going to be like this, but now I see it's like that instead. Then you can choose to be happy with what is, rather than bemoaning your unrealized fantasies.

Remember That Perspective Is Everything

One day you love your spouse, your kids, your job is good; the next day you can't stand any of them. Why? Nothing has changed but your outlook. The reason could be anything—you're overtired, working too hard, someone did something annoying. It's times like these when we need to keep our perspective, to remember that while we might be feeling completely negative right now, that doesn't necessarily reflect the true range of our experience.

When I get into this state, I say to myself, "I reserve judgment until tomorrow." Chances are I wake up in a much more positive frame of mind. If the discontent persists, I need to look further. Is there something truly terrible going on? Is there a problem we need to work out? Do I need to talk with someone else and get an outside opinion? By keeping our perspective, we prevent little bumps in the road from turning into gaping potholes. Is there an issue you could use a little perspective on right now?

Give Yourself a Boys' (or Girls') Night Out

My husband gets together with a group of five other guys once a month to play poker. They've been playing together for fifteen years. They take turns making dinner and hosting the event, and he never makes it home before 2 A.M. I used to turn my nose up at it, but I've come to see that it is a chance for them not only to have fun, but to keep connected to one another. They've been there for their marriages, births of babies, work changes, relationship breakups. But the main point is to have fun, and what's wrong with that?

Sometimes we all need to go out, stay up late, and kick up our heels. When was the last time you did something like that?

Receive a "Scent"sational Break

Take your favorite essential oil (peach, rose, and vanilla are all nice environmental scents), and rub it on the light bulbs in your bedroom before you turn them on this evening. The room will be infused with scent as the light heats up the oil. Yum!

Expect the Best

Moods tend to generalize. What I mean by that is that you can get on a roll of feeling bad and carry it over day after day till suddenly a month has gone by with you in a gray fog.

We can stop such a cycle, however, when we remember that every day is a new one and that we should expect the best today no matter what. As Iyanla Vanzant remembers in *Yesterday I Cried*, her spiritual teacher once said, "Just because it rained yesterday and the ground is flooded, that does not mean you are going to get wet today."

Try adopting that as your slogan for today.

You Can't Do It Alone

Over and over research has shown that feelings of loneliness and isolation are major impediments to a happy and healthy life. We really do need one another, and the more we cut ourselves off from others, the more unhappy we will be. And the more we try to bring happiness into other people's lives, the more we will experience it ourselves. The problem is that when we feel bad, many of us (me included) have the tendency to isolate, to crawl into bed and tune out the world.

Sometimes introspection is important, but if you find that you haven't been meeting friends, engaging in meaningful conversations, spending time with those you care about, perhaps you need to push yourself a bit. You can't be happy on your own forever.

Embrace Your Essential Nature

In their wonderful book *True Work,* Michael and Justine Toms tell a great story about an acorn who wants to become a redwood tree. No matter how many positive affirmations the acorn says, no matter how many self-help seminars or diets it tries, it will grow up to be an oak, not a redwood. "Enormous power and strength is available when you act from your essential nature," they remind us. And to power and strength, I would add happiness too.

Embracing our essence is not necessarily easy. For many of us, our essence is so intrinsic as to be invisible; to others it is devalued because it feels so ordinary—we keep thinking it's *better* to be a redwood than an oak. In my twenties, I used to believe that I wasn't "supposed" to be an editor because it was too easy for me. And, until my forties, I thought that while I was an essentially solitary, early-to-bed bookworm, any day I could turn into a wild extrovert who partied all night if I wanted to.

If your essence eludes you, ask a friend, "When you think of me, what adjectives come to mind?" Ask yourself, "When do I feel most true to myself?"

Have a Makeover

This is another feel-good, absolutely free mood elevator. Just go to any large department store and cruise the makeup counters. Choose someone to make you over. Perhaps you'll end up liking how you look so much that you buy some skin and beauty products. But you can have fun playing regardless. (I also love to go to the wig section and see how I'd look in various hair colors and styles—I make a hideous blonde.)

Trust Your Happiness

Do you, somewhere in the dark recesses of your heart, believe that you don't deserve to be happy? Or that you can't trust happiness because the universe is an unfriendly place out to get you? Is it difficult for you to appreciate what you have because you're afraid of losing it?

The truth is that no one deserves to be happy more than you. And happiness is available to each of us in every single moment, no matter what else is happening, if we just make a commitment to it over and over again.

Trust in happiness and you will experience an everflowing stream.

Reconnect with an Old Friend

Jenny, who works with me, told me the other day about how much pleasure she got from looking up an old friend. "We hadn't spoken in fifteen years, but I just got it into my head that I wanted to touch base. I tracked him down and we played phone tag for a while, but last night we spoke. We had such a good time catching up on mutual friends, kids, and what's been going on in our own lives."

There isn't anything quite like the pleasure of reconnection, is there? Who might you like to reconnect with?

Revision Work

Sometimes we need to shake up the way we work because we've become stagnant and therefore bored. Here's a wonderful suggestion on how to de-stagnate from Paul Pearsall in *Write Your Own Pleasure Prescription*. He calls it a "wondering about work" list:

"Write down three ways that you could do your job differently and still get done what you have to do. Consider anything that might be allowed where you work, such as playing different music every day, changing your time of arrival or departure, or working on the weekend and taking a day off during the week. Ask yourself what it is that might make your work an avocation instead of a vocation."

Unwind with Chamomile

Chamomile is considered an antidepressant that is also a mild sleep aid. So here's a wonderful way to relax before going to sleep. Make a cup of chamomile tea, and then run a warm bath. Add two chamomile tea bags to the bath water. Bring your cup of tea, along with a pen and pad of paper with you into the tub. As you sip, make a list of ten wishes you want to come true in your life. Sleep well!

Pump Iron

It has been proven again and again that exercise can raise our spirits. But recently a study has shown that of all types of exercise you can do, lifting weights lifts your spirits the most. Scientists at Arizona State University studied the effects of different kind of exercise on the moods of folks sixty-two and older. By far, weight training worked the best. One theory as to why is that the benefits come quickly. Most people can increase their weight limit by five pounds in only a week, whereas the progress in other forms of exercise is slower.

You don't even need to purchase official weights. One friend lifts rocks of similar weight that she found on the beach.

Oh, Well

This one I learned from my two-year-old. Whenever she loses something or something breaks or goes wrong, she says in her most cheery voice, "Oh, well." Oh well, my favorite seashell broke. Oh well, I can't find my favorite book *Goodnight Moon*. Oh well, we have no more cranberry juice.

Ana says it not resignedly, not bitterly, but from that perfectly philosophical place that recognizes that whatever has happened is no big deal: that pain comes from trying to cling to things that are absolutely definitely going to disappear at some point, and that happiness is found in flowing with what is, rather than wishing it were different. Sometimes I wonder if she comes by this wisdom innately, or whether it is a product of her early life. Abandoned on a street at birth, left lying in a crib with virtually no attention for a year, she already knows what's important—and what's not. To Ana, the love she can give and receive today matters; the fact that her pink rabbit's gone missing does not. I only wish I could be as wise.

"Oh, well" is such a wonderful practice in nonattachment. It helps us to remember that most of what we are upset about really doesn't matter. What do you need to say "Oh, well" about today?

Don't Take It Personally

Oh, this one is so hard for me! But the truth is that life is full of both wonderful and terrible things. Both happen for no apparent reason, but naturally we find something challenging harder to take—cancer strikes despite the fact that you have taken good care of yourself; the company for which you've worked for thirty years takes its manufacturing overseas and you're out of a job; your house is struck by lightning and burns to the ground.

Bad things happen that are beyond our control, but we add to our reasonable unhappiness over a difficult circumstance by taking it personally. We feel our bosses were out to get us specifically. Or that if only we had done something different, the terrible thing would not have occurred. I think what really happens in these situations is that we come face to face with how uncontrollable and unpredictable so much of life truly is, and rather than surrendering control, which is scary, we'd rather fix blame on ourselves or someone else.

Right now, we are all living through social, economic, and technological changes of unprecedented proportions. We need to swim in this fast-moving river as best we can, trying to keep our heads above water, not torment ourselves by taking the challenges personally.

Be a Johnny Tulipbulb

Plant a few bulbs in some public place: the median strip outside your office, the corner of the park down the street, the edge of the office parking lot. You'll have fun now thinking of next spring when they suddenly burst into color.

Ferret Out a Bargain

I love to save money—it never fails to give me a boost: the $50 sweater I got for $20, the two packages of pasta for the price of one at Safeway. I thought this form of happiness was particular to my penny-pinching New England soul, but the more I spoke to people about this book, the more I saw that many folks share my pleasure in saving money. My latest discovery is consignment shopping—other people's "gently used" and usually designer clothes at a fraction of the retail price.

So, get out there a score a bargain!

Do a Good Deed for Someone You Know

This is like a random act of kindness, except it's not random. For no reason, do something nice for someone you know. Do a chore that is usually your spouse's responsibility (one that he or she hates will be particularly appreciated). Bring in a flower for everyone in your office or team. Offer to make a special dinner for a friend recovering from surgery. Bake your children's favorite cake. The more we create joy for others, the more we'll feel it in ourselves.

Throw a Joy Party

Call or send invitations to those who seem like good happiness teachers in your life. Invite them to a party in which you'll not only enjoy one another's company, but each person will have the chance to talk about what brings them happiness and joy. Suggest that guests might want to bring something inspirational to read, or an uplifting piece of music to share. Serve a wonderful meal and share your words of wisdom. Go around the table and ask people to talk about the happiest moment of their lives, and what they've learned about living with joy.

Spritz Up

Here's a wonderful pick-me-up that uses one of my favorite scents—bergamot. Bergamot is a light, flowery essential oil that is a mood lifter. All you need is a small plastic spray bottle. Make a body spray by combining 1 cup of water with 2 drops of lavender essential oil and 2 drops bergamot. Shake well and spray on hands and face any time you need a boost.

Look Deeply at Someone You Love

When we fall in love with someone, we spend a lot of time gazing at him or her, memorizing every little laugh wrinkle, the curve of his lips, the golden flecks in her brown eyes. Over time, however, our senses get jaded, and we no longer truly *see* the amazing being right in front of our eyes.

When we lose someone we love, often a big regret is that we didn't appreciate the person enough. If only we could gaze into those golden eyes one more time, hear that tinkly laughter once more.

Right now, while you still can, really look at the person you love. Don't miss this chance to drink him or her in.

Map Your Support System

It's easy to feel isolated, as if you are completely alone in the world. The truth is we all have a personal support system, and by becoming more aware of ours, we can feel more secure.

Get a large piece of paper. Draw a circle in the center to represent yourself. Then, radiating out from the circle, draw smaller circles to represent the members of your support network. They may be fellow church members, coworkers, therapists, ministers, neighbors, family members—anyone whom you can count on for assistance of any kind. Write down their name in the circle and the kind of support they give—listening, financial support, rides, baby-sitting, whatever.

Now step back and look at the picture as a whole. Take in the fact that you are supported, that you have others you can count on. Are there areas where you could use a bit more help? Are you relying too much on one or two people? Should you extend your network?

Refurbish a Piece of Furniture

Because so many of us work primarily with our heads, doing something with our hands can provide a tremendous sense of satisfaction. I have an old pine blanket chest that I bought about twenty years ago. Over the years it has endured dog scratches, children's scribbles, and scrapes from candleholders. I looked at it recently and thought, "It needs some help." So I sanded it down a bit, and applied coat after coat of Briwax and then cream furniture polish. Now it glows again, and I smile every time I walk into the room.

One way to experience this good feeling is to find something with intrinsic quality and value. If someone once cared about the piece and put quality in, no matter how many layers of paint and neglect followed, you can restore it. Enjoy the sense of creativity and preserving the past.

Or do what my coworker Brenda does. Find a junky wooden or metal chair that is being thrown away, and save it from the landfill. Use your imagination and paint it to have a one-of-a-kind creation. Each leg a different color? The sky on the seat? Go wild.

Go Out for Breakfast

My father was an old-fashioned country doctor who made house calls and visited his patients in the county hospital every day of the week except Sunday. On Saturdays, he would get up early and, on the way to the hospital, stop for breakfast at what my mother always referred to as "the dirty diner." It was a greasy spoon in an old railroad car with split black leather booths. Its chief appeal was the break it provided in his routine of coffee and the newspaper before rushing off to work.

OCTOBER

9

Neither am I a regular breakfast eater, but like him, I have learned the pleasure of a regular breakfast out. It's a chance to slow down and observe the start of the day through new eyes. Plus, eating breakfast has been shown to be good for you both mentally and physically, as long as you don't have bacon and eggs daily.

So go to a diner or café and sit among people you normally don't see. You can still read the newspaper, but remember to listen to new sounds and conversation and enjoy the smells that only breakfast produces.

Take in Touch

Why do you walk through the fields in gloves when the grass is soft as the breasts of doves and shivering sweet to the touch?
—Frances Cornford

We touch so many things in the course of a day, but do we really *feel* anything? Our sense of touch is one of the miracles of our bodies that we often grow numb to. When I was a kid, I knew a boy who had a disease that caused him to be numb all over. He could move, but he couldn't feel anything—hot or cold, wet or dry, nothing. I remember vividly when I met him how much his suffering—he kept getting hurt because he had no warning system—reminded me of the preciousness of my sense of touch.

Take a few moments right now to really feel something. Scratch your belly with awareness, or feel the little hairs on your arm. Notice how touch has two components—the sensation in your fingertips and the sensations your fingertips create on your skin. Revel in your ability to feel. Isn't that great?

A Recipe for True Contentment

According to *Awakening the Buddha Within*, Buddha once said that happiness is created by four things: "to be skilled, efficient, earnest, and learned in whatever profession one has; to conscientiously protect one's income and family's means of support; to have virtuous, trustworthy, and faithful friends and spiritual aspirations; to be content and live within one's means."

Take a few moments to think about your life. Are these things true for you? Where might you need more work? For each of us the answer is different, but unless we are "on path" with all four, our lives will most likely not be happy.

Create Happiness around You

I was reading some e-mails that had been forwarded to me today and came across a letter from a man named Larry Harp. He reflected on the priorities in his life, now that we are at the new millennium. One of them was, "I want [people] to be happier when I come into a room than when I leave."

What a fabulous priority. I'm going to make it my pledge for the day. I'm not sure how I will do it, but I will keep the thought in the foreground of my consciousness and see what happens. How about you?

Learn Something from an Elder

The world is changing so fast, and much of what the generations who came before us knew, appreciated, and experienced is in danger of being lost forever. But the more the future takes us into the unknown, the more the past, particularly the past of our families, is valuable. (That's why, I believe, that the study of genealogy is currently the biggest leisure pastime in the United States). Wisdom, the learning that life offers about what matters most, is timeless and priceless in this information-overloaded society.

Today, make a date with an older relative to learn about his upbringing, immigration story, traditions. Ask about the most important lessons she's learned. Ask him how he dealt with grief and loss, about the most significant event in her life. It will enrich your life and make him or her feel valued.

A Year to Live

When I was studying gratitude for *Attitudes of Gratitude,* I was struck again and again by the fact that the most grateful people seemed to be those who had had a brush with death. Somehow it takes facing our mortality to wake us up to the beauty of simply being alive.

This is so powerful that entire books have been written on how imagining that you have only a year to live wakes you up to what really matters in your life and increases your happiness in the present moment. Stephen Levine's book *A Year to Live* takes you step by step through the whole year as you prepare to "die."

To get a sense of what this can do for your attitude, try this: Imagine you are going to die one year from today. Write down what you would do between now and then. Who would you spend time with? Where would you go? How would you act differently? What legacy would you want to leave?

Now look at your list and notice the difference between it and how you are living right now. Pick just one thing and schedule it in your appointment book right now.

Get Out Your Camera

When kids are little, it's easy to take lots of pictures. Kids are so cute, you want to record every stage. But I was surprised recently to go through old photo albums and realize that, aside from kid photos, all my pictures were of exotic places I've been to. I had virtually none of the people who I care about the most—my friends, my sister—and none of the places I've lived.

Why wait for the trip to Hawaii? How about getting out your camera and taking some pictures of your everyday surroundings—your office, the black poppy blooming in your garden, the friends coming over for dinner? Take some time to record what's around you day to day and learn to look at it from new angles and perspectives. And you'll have a wonderful record to go back to later, when your life is different.

The Water Meditation

All you need is water to try this meditation from *Awakening the Buddha Within* by Lama Surya Das—a stream, a pool, even a sink of dishes:

"Listen to the 'white sound' of water. Enter into the contemplative space, the flow, the reflectiveness of water. Concentrate on the sound of water. Let it wash everything else away. . . . Enter the resonant spiritual dimension of pure sound.

"Open your eyes. Look at the water. Let all thoughts fall into the water and dissolve into the lake of your mind, like snowflakes settling and dissolving in the ocean. All waves of thought and feeling, and emotion and energy, gradually slow down and dissolve, like gentle ripples in a stream in the placid sea of natural awareness. . . .

"Be that sound, flow with the water. Relax into the natural state of the water element as if worshipping the spirit of nature or the deity of water. . . . Enter into that sacred dimension now."

The Joke's on Them

Humor is so personal—what one person might find funny another might think stupid or even insensitive. I am not generally known as a particularly funny person, but two friends think I'm hilarious; our funny bones just happen to match.

Now there is an online joke service designed by researchers at the University of California at Berkeley that claims to be able to evaluate your humor preferences. Log on to **http.//shadow.ieor.berkeley.edu/humor**. There you will read ten jokes, which you rank on a sliding scale. Then you'll receive a series of knee slappers sure to make you laugh. Or so they say.

Come to the Banquet

Today's the day to emulate Auntie Mame, "the queen of abundant living," as Sue Patton Thoele calls her. Mame grabbed all the juice she could out of life, proclaiming, "Life's a banquet and some poor fools are starving to death!"

We can all experience such exuberance if we just give ourselves permission. What can you do to pull up a chair to the banquet of life? Splurge on a new dress? Roll naked in the grass? Go dancing? Go to a playground and swing on the swings?

Soak Your Feet

Indulge yourself with a foot soak. All you need are a large bowl, your favorite essential oil, two handfuls or so of marbles (you'll see), some rose petals (optional), and a pumice stone. Mix a few drops of the essential oil in the bowl and fill with warm water. Drop the marbles in carefully and float the flower petals. Place your feet in the bowl and use the marbles as a massage tool. Soak five to ten minutes. Remove your feet from the water, and use pumice on the rough spots. Dry your feet and massage with a foot cream. Heavenly!

Make Your Bed

This is a tough one for me. I have never made my bed, at least not since I left home. And as a child it was one of the major bones of contention between my mother and me.

But it is a happiness creator—studies show that making your bed in the morning can keep depression away. Maybe because it gives the maker a sense of accomplishment—no matter what else happens in this day, at least the bed is made. It's like a period at the end of a sentence—now you're ready to begin the day. And coming back in the evening to a crisply made bed will give you a bonus lift.

Discover Something New
about a Friend

Just like love relationships, friendships can get into ruts. We can spend a great deal of time with our friends and not know very much about what really matters to them.

There are all kinds of ways to deepen a relationship. One easy one is to try asking hypothetical questions (Would you rather become deaf or blind and why?; What would you do if . . . ?) that reveal a side you've never seen before.

Or you can ask a friend to tell you what has been the most significant lesson they've learned in life and how they learned it. Or ask them to tell you a recent dream they had. Or which parent they're closer to and why. The point is to get off the surface level and deepen the encounter. Merely by intending it you'll find the way.

Notice the Half-Full Glass

This is standard advice to pessimists. Instead of noticing all of what's wrong, cheer yourself up by focusing on what's right in your life. Train yourself to notice that the glass is half-full instead of half-empty, and you will be happier no matter what is going on.

It's easy to say, and as a recovering pessimist, I can testify that it is possible to retrain yourself to look on the positive side.

Recently I read a new spin on that idea from bestselling author Iyanla Vanzant. She is an inspiring example of someone who has turned her life around from extreme hardship to phenomenal success. She reminds us that "no matter how much is in the glass, it is for that time, in that moment, as full as it's going to get." The key words here are *in that moment*. Right now, for each of us, the glass is as full as it is going to get. That says nothing about tomorrow, or next week. Just right now. So enjoy however full it might be.

You Are My Other Self

I recently read a piece about the Toltecs, a group of Indians living primarily in Mexico. Their traditional greeting when meeting another person is, "You are my other self." What a beautiful sentiment! To understand so profoundly the truth of our connection.

What would it mean for you to go through your day figuratively greeting each person that way? How would your response to them be different? How would you feel?

Turn Down the Lights

As much as we have distanced ourselves from nature, the truth is that we are still biological creatures who are subject to the laws of nature. Nowhere is this more true than with our sleep patterns (that's why I hate the switch from Daylight Savings Time and back again—it's not natural to jerk our bodies around like that).

Our biological clocks are so regulated by changes in light and darkness that, according to Margaret Moline, director of the Sleep-Wake Disorders Center at the New York Hospital, even fifteen minutes of bright light can inhibit your ability to go to sleep.

So if you have trouble falling asleep, be sure to keep the lights low in the evening—use candles, dimmers, lamps. Not only is low lighting flattering and romantic, it will help you get the shut-eye you need to be energetic and feel great.

Let Go of Outcome

So much of what happens to us is out of our control. All we can do is set our intentions and be willing to dance with whatever happens, navigating according to the compass of our deepest values, continuing to move to the place of greatest possibility.

Unfortunately, most of us haven't been taught well how to do this. We get attached to results and then are disappointed when it doesn't turn out the way we expected or hoped. We get attached to the past, wishing and hoping that things could go back to the way they used to be. Both attitudes are prescriptions for misery.

Letting go of the outcome doesn't mean that we don't work toward something. Just that if it doesn't happen, we don't take it personally, but rather readjust to the new reality. Here's an example: In the process of adopting a child, I met many couples who were obsessed with having a biological child and had spent thousands of dollars trying. If their intention was to have a child, at some point they needed to say, "I guess this is not going to turn out the way we thought. Let's consider adoption." Those who made that leap ended up very happy. Those who could not ended up with a hole in their lives. Is there an expected outcome in your life right now that you need to let go of and accept things as they are?

Try Some Candle Magic

How about conjuring up your heart's desire with candle magic? Writes Margie Lapanja in *Goddess in the Kitchen*, "Candles have been employed in almost every religious and spiritual tradition since fire was discovered. The flame symbolizes the energy of intention that is both released and attracted, and the light of the flame guides and illuminates these desires. The dripping wax represents the grounding power of the earth, while the dance of the flame resonates with the energy of manifestation.... Let me add one vital note: Be careful of what you ask for because, if you have faith, you'll get it."

In candle magic, the color of the candle symbolizes what you wish to manifest:

Red: love, passion, courage; *Orange:* concentration, emotional stability, healthy sexuality; *Yellow:* creativity; *Green:* abundance, health; *Sky blue:* peace, intuition; *Dark blue:* protection; *Purple:* power; *White:* purification, clarity; *Pink:* honor, friendship, happiness; *Silver:* serenity; *Black:* release.

Be sure to make sure you use sturdy candleholders, and never leave a flame unattended.

Make Use of Whatever Happens to You

*There is only one group of people that don't have prob-
lems and they're all dead. Problems are a sign of life. So
the more problems you have the more alive you are.*
—Norman Vincent Peale

OCTOBER

27

As the late great minister points out, problems are
endemic to the human condition. No one escapes. The
trick is to use whatever problem, difficulty, or hardship
you are facing as a vehicle for spiritual and emotional
growth. It isn't always easy, and it isn't always possible to
do in the moment, but there are always hidden blessings in
difficult situations, and when we discover them, we
redeem our suffering. We make meaning out of tragedy
and grow more loving, compassionate, patient, and kind
as a consequence.

The people I admire most all say that they are grateful
for the hard things they faced because of these opportunities for growth: a heart attack that reconnected them to
their feelings, cancer that forced them to slow down,
financial difficulties that taught them resilience.

Think about the most challenging thing you are facing
right now. How is it an opportunity for you to grow your
soul?

Consider Sammy

The use of St. John's Wort as a natural alternative to Prozac is well known, but recently another supplement has come along that rivals St. John in effectiveness: S-adebosylme-thionine, commonly known as "Sammy." Sammy is a natural compound found in people and in animals and has been used in Europe for more than twenty years to treat mild depression. It has no known side effects and usually works within a week (as opposed to St. John's Wort, which can take up to six weeks to kick in). The drawbacks? It's very expensive—$25 for twenty capsules (check out the discount online pharmacies listed in the reading for March 5), and it is not recommended for people who suffer from bipolar disorders, because it can increase mania. Doctors are also worried that it will encourage those with serious depression to avoid getting the professional help they need. Check with your doctor before self-medicating.

Take in a Matinee

When was the last time you went to a movie in the middle of the day? Go ahead, indulge yourself. If you're feeling particularly daring, see a double feature. And don't forget to get a big bucket of popcorn and a box of your favorite candy.

Cultivate the Positive

Happiness, teaches the Dalai Lama and other great sages, comes from cultivating positive states of mind and eliminating negative ones. What that means is to experience as much as possible generosity, compassion, tolerance, and patience toward ourselves and others. When anger, fear, anxiety, or hatred arise in us (the enemies of happiness, say the Buddhists), we need to use our capacity for generosity, compassion, tolerance, and patience to eliminate them.

This is a lifelong work. For today, it is enough to commit to cultivating generosity, compassion, tolerance, and patience. When we dedicate ourselves to practicing these positive states, we take a giant leap toward bringing them into our lives on a daily basis.

Create an Adventure

This is most easily done on a weekend, but if you're up to playing hooky, that makes it all the more enjoyable. Kidnap a friend or loved one, and take him or her on an adventure in which he or she has no idea where you are going and you are totally in charge. Have a picnic by a lake, take in a country fair, go to an amusement park—whatever you and the other person will enjoy. Include a number of surprises during the day—a new bathing suit for the swimming portion of the trip, a necklace to wear for dinner, a series of notes for a treasure hunt. Be as creative as you can. You'll have the joy of planning and seeing your loved one's reaction; he or she will have the thrill of a surprise.

Make a Place to Rest Your Eyes

You can put this at home or at the office, anywhere you need a restful place. Nothing could be easier than this Zen centerpiece; it will foster serenity anywhere. Find or buy small dark rocks of uniform size. Rinse them in a colander. Take an attractive shallow bowl and fill the bottom with one or two inches of rocks, depending on the depth of the container—you're creating a rock bottom. Fill with water up to one inch from the top rim. Place a candle or two and a blossom such as a gardenia or hibiscus in the water, and allow them to float.

Relive a Happy Moment

Today is the Day of the Dead, celebrated in Mexico as the time in which all those who have passed on come back and celebrate with the living. In honor of the occasion, take a moment to remember a happy memory of your loved ones who have passed on. I remember a game I would play with my father. He would be in the bathroom with the door closed. I must have been five or so. I would knock and he would sing the old song, "Who's That Knocking at My Door?" and pretend he didn't know me. I would howl with laughter.

What happy memory pops into your mind when you think of a loved one who has died? Relive it now.

Revitalize Instantly

One theory why so many of us are dragging around and feeling listless is that we are all suffering from B-complex vitamin deficiency. In *Natural Energy Boosters,* Carlson Wade suggests that the best and quickest way to replenish our store of B-vitamins is with brewer's yeast. He claims a shot of brewer's yeast when you're feeling lowly will beat tiredness, increase energy, and help resist depression.

Try his "Instant Pep Tonic"—½ teaspoonful of brewer's yeast added to any fresh fruit or vegetable juice. Add a bit of honey for flavoring, if desired. Stir vigorously or process in the blender. Drink slowly. If you find this tonic helps, you might want to consider bringing a jar of brewer's yeast to the office for those afternoon energy lags.

Act On an Inner Impulse

Young kids are so spontaneous. If they feel like doing somersaults, they do. If they want to run around in circles, they do. However, they are quickly taught to conform, to curb their impulses and fit in, and by the time they are adults virtually all of their spontaneity is completely hidden.

Right now, just for a moment, experience again the exuberance of childhood by following one of your inner impulses. It could be anything—whatever comes into your mind. Whoop out loud? Rip off your tie and skip across the room? Stretch like a cat? Whatever it is, give yourself permission to do it.

It Doesn't Have to Be Hard

Where did so many of us get the idea if we are too happy, something terrible is going to happen? We can't enjoy ourselves, can't let our guard down because we think that being hypervigilant will protect us. It's magical thinking to believe that we can ward off disaster by not being too happy. As the great philosopher Epictetus reminds us, "When considering the future, remember that all situations unfold as they do regardless of how we feel about them." We can exercise caution and care, we can plan and scheme, but to a great extent, life unfolds on a grander scale than all our scheming. Worry will do nothing to change the outcome.

It doesn't have to be hard. It's OK if it is easy.

Recognize Your Magnificence

My father had a healthy sense of self-esteem (he helped me gain one too). No false modesty for him—he would revel in his fine mind and his beautiful silver hair. What kept him from being conceited was that he felt equally as strongly about everyone else he came across—he noticed and celebrated other people's unique magnificence as well.

From him I learned that it is not only OK but wonderful to celebrate yourself. You are the only you, an irreplaceable, unreplicable being of light and love. Tell yourself five great things about yourself as you wake up today (or go to sleep tonight).

Say You're Sorry

Apologizing is one of the greatest happiness acts we can do, and so many of us are resistant. We got the idea that saying sorry will cause us to lose face or power or something, and we stubbornly stick to our guns and the distance between us and the other person grows.

My husband, Don, taught me about the beauty of apology. He has no resistance to it whatsoever. If I say I'm hurt by him in any way, he says, "I'm sorry." And because of his shining example, I find it easy to apologize now too. You can't imagine how many hours of fighting we've avoided as a result! We don't need to fight about most things because we don't have to convince the other that we've been injured.

Defensiveness keeps us disconnected from one another. Next time someone says you've hurt them, try the two magic words, *I'm sorry.*

Find a Fun Lunch Spot

Going out to lunch creates a wonderful work break, but it's easy to get stuck running yet again to the corner deli. In my poll of happiness boosters, several people mentioned the pleasurable thrill they get when they find a good new lunch spot.

So break your routine and put some variety into your diet. Seek out a hot new spot.

Splurge on Childhood Delights

Eating is not merely a material pleasure. Eating gives a spectacular joy to life and contributes immensely to good-will and happy companionship.
—Elsa Schiaperelli

What is your favorite food memory from childhood? Mine is my grandmother's fudge and her mustard pickles (not eaten together, thank you). I haven't had either in years.

Chances are you haven't indulged in your nursery favorite either, but maybe today is the time to splurge. Do you have the recipes? If not, can you call a relative and track them down? Or try looking in *Square Meals* by Jane and Michael Stern, or *Best Recipes from the Backs of Boxes, Bottles, Cans and Jars* by Ceil Dyer. Your great-aunt Tilly's world famous potato salad may have been from the Best mayonnaise jar. My grandma's one-of-a-kind fudge is still printed on jars of Marshmallow Fluff.

Folk Cures for the Blues

Try the pizza cure. Eat it or any other food with lots of oregano. Oregano is believed to relieve that heavy-hearted feeling associated with depression.

Or try two ripe bananas. Bananas contain both norepinephrine and serotonin, which are antidepressants.

If you have a juicer, try a combination of half-spinach and half-watercress juice. If you can't stand the taste, throw in a carrot. The blend is said to raise your spirits.

Green Cheer

A green plant is a wonderful happiness booster. One of the hardiest and easiest to grow plants is a sweet potato. Even if you consider yourself to have a black thumb, try this—it grows fast and it's almost impossible to kill. (OK, you do have to keep the glass full of water, but that's it.)

All you do is get an old glass jar (a cleaned-out spaghetti sauce jar is just right) and fill it with water. Buy a sweet potato at the grocery store and poke four toothpicks in the center as if you were marking the four directions (north, south, east, and west), and place the bottom half of the sweet potato in the water. (The toothpicks will keep the whole potato from being submerged.) Place in a sunny window and wait, adding water if necessary. Soon you'll have graceful vines and big curving leaves crawling all over the sill.

What Are You Here For?

It's so easy to get wrapped up in the ups and downs of our individual lives that we forget that we are really here to serve. How can you begin to offer your unique gifts to the world? How can you better use the gifts you've been given?

To serve is to find our highest purpose and to be used to our fullest. What could be better than that? As Albert Schweitzer reminds us, "I don't know what your destiny will be, but one thing I do know: the only ones among you who will be really happy are those who have sought and found how to serve."

Here's a way to discover your purpose, described by Sanaya Roman in *Living with Joy:* "Close your eyes and allow a picture, symbol or image to come to mind that represents your purpose here on earth. Bring your symbol into your heart. Ask the higher forces of the universe to breathe more light and life into it. Draw your symbol. . . . Imagine your symbol changing color, texture and size, and let it speak to you with its wisdom and show you how it can be released to help serve mankind."

Speak Your Truth

Family therapists know that there is a surefire formula for disaster in any relationship: withhold, withdraw, project. This means that if we keep something significant from a person with whom we are in a relationship—how we feel or what we are thinking—we naturally begin to withdraw from that person. And when we withdraw, it's then easy to project all kinds of negative things on the other person because we aren't having a true back-and-forth. And that causes a great deal of unhappiness for both. Here's an example of what I mean: I am angry at you, but am afraid to say so. So I withdraw. Suddenly everything you do seems to drive me crazy. I imagine all kinds of bad motivations for your behavior, and our relationship deteriorates.

Is there someone in your life from whom you've withdrawn because you are withholding something? I encourage you to have the courage to express it, verbally or in writing. You can do it kindly. Even if it is something that might be difficult for the two of you to go through, sharing it will ultimately lead to greater connection and happiness.

Read Out Loud

We read aloud to little kids, but why do we tend to stop as they get older? It's a wonderful way for parents and kids of all ages and couples to spend time together.

I have friends who take turns reading *The Hobbit* to one another for half an hour before they go to sleep. It's a way of connecting that doesn't require conversation, but promotes delight and intimacy. They look forward each night to climbing into bed.

If you're not up to a whole book, why not find a passage that you love and read it aloud to someone tonight?

Write a Fan Note

One of the most wonderful surprises I had in recent years was receiving a note from Sue Bender, author of the best-selling books *Plain and Simple* and *Everyday Sacred*. She had heard me speak at a publishing seminar and wrote to me out of the blue to say how much she appreciated my spirit. What an incredible gift!

Is there someone you've met recently who impressed you? Let them know. Send an e-mail or make a phone call. Perhaps it is a coworker whose steadfastness or ingenuity has always struck you. Or a neighbor whose flower garden never fails to lift your mood. The trick here is to send a message to someone who is either a stranger—as in my case—or someone who doesn't know you well and is therefore not expecting anything from you.

Mind Cleaner

So many of us do mental work. It's easy for our minds to get tired, to be drained of all creativity and joy. If your mind needs a boost, try this Austrian remedy for mental fatigue.

Core and cut a washed apple into very small pieces and place in a bowl. Pour 2 cups of boiling water over the apple and let sit for one hour. Add 1 tablespoon honey and stir. Drink the liquid and eat the apple.

Create a Love Gallery

Years ago, my husband and I started hanging pictures of loved ones up on a wall in our living room. They never failed to give me a lift as I walked in the door at the end of the day. We've moved several times, but our photo gallery always goes with us—hallways are a particularly good place for such photos.

If you don't want to go to the trouble of framing photos (we buy inexpensive black frames to create visual harmony), you can simply tack photos onto a bulletin board or attach them to the fridge with magnets. Any place where they will bring a smile to your lips.

Appreciate This Present Moment

This one. Right now. It's so easy to forget. As Thich Nhat Hanh says, "We know how to sacrifice ten years for a diploma, and we are willing to work very hard to get a job, a car, a house, and so on. But we have difficulty remembering that we are alive in the present moment, the only moment there is for us to be alive. Every breath we take, every step we make, can be filled with peace, joy, and serenity. We need only to be awake, alive in the present moment."

This one.

Create Holiday Potpourri

Here's a great mixture you can make for Thanksgiving or the end of the year holidays, to give as gifts to teachers, to bring to open houses or other holiday get-togethers. The smell is guaranteed to lift your heart.

Combine 1 cup whole allspice, 1 cup star anise, 1 cup sliced fresh ginger, 2 cups sliced orange peel, 2 cups dried rose petals, and 2 cups lemon verbena leaves in a clean, dry glass jar with a lid. Add 30 drops allspice essential oil, 5 drops at a time, combining well after each addition. Store in a covered jar or, if you want to give as gifts, package in plastic bags or small jars.

To use, pour ⅔ cup into 2–3 cups water and simmer gently on the stove to release aroma. You can reheat this until odor is gone.

King or Queen for an Hour

Here's a wonderful idea for any two family members, but especially a couple, from Jennifer Louden's *The Couple's Comfort Book:*

"Flip a coin to see who will go first. The partner who wins the coin toss rules for the next hour. Agree ahead of time that no request is out of bounds; the person of the hour is to be treated to whatever he or she wishes. When the hour is up (use a timer), the next person is crowned for his or her hour of royalty."

Try a Relaxing Breath

There are many breathing techniques, each designed to do something different. Some are energizing; others are relaxing. Here is one derived from yoga that Dr. Andrew Weil swears by for relaxing. He recommends it for falling asleep, going back to sleep after being awakened, or when you are feeling angry or upset.

Lie or sit comfortably. Touch the tip of your tongue to the ridge of tissue on the roof of your mouth behind your upper front teeth. Exhale completely through the mouth to the count of eight, making a *whooo* sound. Inhale through the nose to the count of four. Hold your breath to the count of seven, then exhale again to the count of eight. Do four complete cycles of inhalation, holding and exhalation, all the while keeping your tongue on the ridge on the roof of your mouth. Then breathe normally.

Be Aware That Your Words Create Reality

It used to be believed that language was a mirror of reality, an attempt to articulate what was already "out there" in the world. But recently, there has been a great deal of research that proves that it actually works the other way—the images we hold of the world and the language we use actually create reality. (My favorite study in this vein was one where teachers were told that particular kids in their class were extremely intelligent; actually they were average. By the end of the year, those kids were at the top of the class. The teachers' belief in their intelligence helped them to *become* smarter!)

We can use this phenomenon to become happier by choosing upbeat rather than negative or neutral words to describe ourselves and our situations. Begin by tracking the words you tend to use to describe yourself and your life. Are they negative, positive, or neutral? Then find positive synonyms for your negative words. Here are some of mine: for *nervous* or *worried*, I substitute *concerned*; for *problem*, use *opportunity*; for *overwhelmed* or *tired*, say *challenged*; for *confused*, try *wondering*.

Allow Thanksgiving
to Bring You Together

The best Thanksgivings I've ever spent are ones in which I feel truly connected to the people I'm with. All too often, however, we're afraid to do the very things that would give us this feeling. But it's not that hard. Here are two simple ideas:

Go around the table, with each person naming one thing they are particularly grateful for this year. Ask each person to talk about who or what has been their greatest teacher and why. Tell a story of how you celebrated Thanksgiving when you were a child.

Or try this: Pass out index cards and ask people to write what they are thankful for in their own lives on one side, and what they appreciate about the other people who are present on the other side. If everyone doesn't know everyone else, have people write thanks for important people who aren't present. Then read your cards before you eat.

Host a Fun Fight

This takes two people. Have a water, shaving cream, or food fight in the kitchen.(It's the easiest place to clean up.) If you're alone with your romantic partner, you might want to try it in the nude.

If you can't stand the idea of a mess, consider a pillow fight instead. The point is to let loose!

Make an Irritation List

This is a way to come into joy through the back door. If you live alone, create a list of all the things that annoy you around the house: the squeaky bedroom door, the dripping faucet, the kitchen drawers that stick. If you live with someone else, make the list together. Prioritize the list—which of all the things would give you the most pleasure if it were fixed? Assign action steps and set a realistic timeframe for completion. Later, you can tackle the rest of the items on the list, one by one.

I promise—fixing even one of these irritating items will bring a smile to your face—as long as you remember to stop and appreciate your work!

Say "Thank You" as Much as Possible

Let's feel the magic of those two little, big words, "thank you."
—Ardath Rodale

In this season of thanksgiving, it's important to remember that consciously saying "Thank you" is the most powerful tool we have to feel instantly joyful. That's because gratitude is the mother of joy. Gratitude makes us feel complete in this moment, full of a sense of well-being that is the experience of joy.

When we say "Thank you" consciously, we anchor in our consciousness that we have been given something, rather than just taking it for granted. At a deeper level, when we acknowledge that we have received something, we acknowledge that we are worthy of being given to, and we build up a positive view of the world as a place in which we are receiving gifts all the time.

So today, try saying "Thank you" for every little thing that is given to you, no matter how small. Look at the giver and really mean it. Notice how you feel at the end of the day.

Imagine Yourself More Competent

In doing the research for this book, I came across a book called *Living with Joy* which is the channeled wisdom of Orin, "a timeless being of love and light," as told to Sanaya Roman. I'm not sure about channeling, but I did like one of Orin's statements: "When you imagine your future, do you not think you will be the same then as you are now." (Timeless beings don't speak in contemporary English, I guess.)

That remark struck me so strongly. I remembered how as each school year approached, I would get increasingly nervous. I'd think to myself, "Yes I got all As in second grade, but third grade is so hard. How will I do it?" Every year I told myself the same story, never remembering that I was growing too, that each year I was older and wiser. I do the same now. I imagine the future as something that I will not be able to cope with, because I envision myself as the same as I am now. I never take further growth into account.

How about you? Take a moment right now to imagine yourself five years from now, with all the wisdom and awareness you'll have gained between now and then. Doesn't it make you feel more secure in the unknown?

Spray the Air

If the dark days of late fall are dragging you down, consider this little pick-me-up—an easy-to-make rose room spray. Besides being the scent of romance, rose is said to have antidepressant properties.

Simply combine 4 drops of rose essential oil, 2 drops of bergamot essential oil, 2 drops of lavender, and 1 cup of water. Place in small plastic spray bottle, shake well, and spray the room.

Take a Success Inventory

It's easy to get focused on failure, on what's hard or not working in our lives. And it's important to look at those things. But it is equally important, and a real mood elevator, to look at how we've succeeded.

Right now, think back over recent days and weeks. What successes, big or small, have you experienced? No fair saying "None." We all do things we can be proud of. What have you done? Did you (finally) have a good conversation with your mother? Get started on that project you've been procrastinating about? Learn to live alone a bit more comfortably? Ran a little extra on your morning jog? Make a list of your successes, and pat yourself on the back.

Compliment a Stranger

I once read a story about a woman who was pulled from her sense of isolation by the mere fact of noticing the Easter outfit an elderly woman was wearing and complimenting her on it. The story stuck with me, and since then I've used it when I want a lift: "That's a great dress you have on," I might say to a person coming toward me at the airport gate. It never fails to make me and the other person smile.

So, as you are walking down the street today, riding in a elevator, standing in line to get a cup of coffee, look around at the people in your general vicinity. Is someone wearing an outrageous hat? Carrying a beautiful bouquet of flowers? Smiling in a particularly charming fashion? Notice something that touches your heart or makes you smile, and comment on it.

Examine What Gets in the Way of Great Holidays

When you think of the six-week period between Thanksgiving and the first of the year, do you look forward to the time with eager anticipation or a sense of dread? For so many of us, the holidays, which can be filled with opportunities for true happiness—a sense of togetherness, a chance to give, a chance to be grateful—are instead occasions for fights, disappointment, overspending, and fatigue.

Today, just take a moment to figure out why the holidays are not happiness enhancers for you. Do you or those around you have unrealistic expectations that you run around trying to fulfill? Do you overspend? Do the holidays bring up feelings of loneliness? Do you have trouble getting along with the relatives that you will spend time with? Today, all you have to do is to identify where the holidays get derailed for you. During the next few weeks, we will look at ways to increase holiday happiness.

Take a Body Break

Just for today, stop thinking of your body as something that must be whipped into shape and notice what you would like to do with it—lie down? Go for a leisurely walk? Make love? Sometimes just giving yourself permission to notice what's true for you can be an amazing way to find happiness—or at least peace of mind.

Oh, to Sleep

Having trouble falling asleep? Consider this natural aromatherapy remedy—a sleep potion made with, among other oils, lavender. Lavender is an adaptogen, which means that it can be stimulating or relaxing, depending on your energy needs. If you are tired, it will help you fall asleep.

In a small plastic spray bottle, combine 4 drops lavender essential oil, 3 drops orange essential oil, 3 drops chamomile essential oil (another good sleep aid), and 5 ounces of water. Shake well. Spray sheets, pillow cases, and the air in your bedroom before sleep.

Consider Nonmaterial Gifts

I once came across a newsletter called *Jumpin' Jan's Flash*. The editor recommended eight wonderful gifts of the spirit to bring happiness to you and your loved ones this year: the gift of listening; the gift of affection; the gift of laughter; the gift of a note of love and appreciation; the gift of a compliment; the gift of a favor; the gift of solitude; the gift of a cheerful disposition.

Would you give one of these gifts today?

Give Gifts That Keep On Giving

This holiday season, make yourself happy by giving presents that matter. All of us have too many sweaters anyway. Great options abound. Here are some ideas to get you started: The Seva Foundation (510-845-7382) helps restore sight to people in India, Nepal, and Tibet and helps indigenous people in Guatemala and Mexico preserve their culture and create sustainable communities; they have a number of very specific gifts that can be given in the name of someone. Ditto the World Vision International Gifts of Joy and Hope (800-423-4200): choose from among things like a goat to a household in Rwanda or literacy training for a child in Bangladesh.

Distract Yourself

Some slight by a friend bugging you? Can't get a coworker's nagging comment out of your mind? A recent study at the University of Michigan shows that dwelling on what's making us mad only increases the intensity of the feeling. Their suggestion—distract yourself.

Get a Massage

We all know that a massage feels good on the outside (as long as whoever is doing it is skilled and sensitive). But it has positive internal effects as well. Massage has been shown to boost the immune system and lower anxiety by reducing cortisol levels (a stress hormone) in the body. There are all kinds of massage; the one you choose is a matter of personal preference.

For the massage to really work—for it to increase pleasure and decrease stress hormones—you need to feel comfortable and relaxed. Some people are concerned about being touched by strangers. If this is true for you, perhaps a friend or loved one can give you a massage, and another day you can return the favor. Remember—this is about your being happy!

Could You Rephrase That, Please?

In the past ten years or so, I've become aware of a terrible habit: I find it extremely difficult in my intimate relationship to ask for something in the positive. Instead of saying, "Would you be so kind as to take out the garbage?" I say, "You never take out the garbage," or, "I hate it when you don't take out the garbage." I have no idea where this comes from, but in trying to break myself of the habit, I have discovered that it is very strong.

I don't think I'm alone. Many of us have trouble asking nicely for what we want and consequently are more unhappy than we need be. Maybe it's because asking directly is so exposing—there's our need right out there on the table for everyone to see and possibly to be ignored or even stomped on. So we come at it sideways or even backward, hoping to get our point across without feeling so vulnerable.

The other people in our lives deserve to be treated nicely. I find that the only thing I can do is think it in the negative and then turn it around in my mind before I speak. When I forget, my husband has learned to ask, "Could you rephrase that, please?"

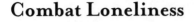

Combat Loneliness

The holiday season can bring on feelings of loneliness, particularly if you are alone or have recently ended a relationship. It's easy to feel that everyone else is having a wonderful time when you are miserable. Here are some coping mechanisms:

1. Consider going away somewhere the holidays are less obvious—perhaps to a cabin in the woods or a Caribbean island.

2. Volunteer at a soup kitchen or homeless shelter. My parents used to do this at Thanksgiving when none of us kids could be there. They felt so good, they weren't lonely.

3. If you've recently broken up, stop yourself from imagining how much fun you'd be having together; remember instead the reasons you ended the relationship.

4. Reach out for support. Call a friend, visit someone, call a hotline.

Unplug Everything

Today, revel in an electronics fast. Imagine the electricity has gone out (and the cellphone too). Let yourself experience a day without faxes, phones, cellphones, e-mail, television, radio. Notice the effect of the fast on your sense of rhythm, your mood, your sense of self-worth, your relationship to others.

Take the Christmas Pledge

It's easy to get caught up in the commercialism of the holidays and overspend and overconsume. When the credit card bills arrive, misery sets in (not to mention you have to live with any children you've spoiled). To avoid such torture and enhance the possibility of holiday happiness, take the Christmas pledge as described in *Unplug the Christmas Machine:* "Believing in the beauty and simplicity of Christmas, I commit to the following: 1. To remember those people who truly need my gifts. 2. To express my love for family and friends in more direct ways than presents. 3. To rededicate myself to the spiritual growth of my family. 4. To examine my holiday activities in light of the true spirit of Christmas. 5. To initiate one act of peacemaking within my circle of family and friends."

Consider Hiring Someone to Help

Sometimes the greatest pleasure can be found in hiring someone to do something for you. Paying someone else to clean the house probably heads people's lists of the most pleasurable outside help we can get. Especially in the hectic holiday season, it can be money well spent!

Make a Love Bouquet

Many of us live far away from those we love most, which can cause sadness at holiday time. Here's a beautiful way to bring faraway loved ones into your celebration, adapted from *The Couple's Comfort Book*. You can do this by yourself or with family members who live with you.

Make a list of those who have been most important to you in your life. Then ask yourself, "If he or she were a flower, what would it be?" Then go to a florist and make a celebration bouquet out of all the flowers that represent your loved ones.

Take a Mental Vacation Today

So much of our daily thoughts and energy go toward worrying about things that never come to pass. Promise yourself, for today, that you'll worry about things tomorrow. It's a great technique when dealing with something over which you have no control. It may not work forever, but it will make you happier today.

Make Holiday Celebrations Easier

For more pleasurable holidays, remember what Susannah Seton says in *Simple Pleasures for the Holidays:* "It's being together that counts. Not how beautiful your tree is, the perfection of your lemon meringue pie, or the spotlessness of your house. . . . The more comfortable and relaxed everyone feels, the more the occasion will be happy. Don't try to do too much—too many activities, too much elaborate food will destroy the fun. And put away things you don't want little ones to ruin—why spend the whole day worrying that Matthew might spill cranberry juice on your white ottoman?"

Today, think about one thing you can do to make your holidays more pleasurable and less stressful. Skip the homemade cards? Have a potluck instead of doing all the work yourself? Get your spouse to wrap the presents?

Give Up Holiday Perfection

I know a woman who is always miserable at holiday time because things never turn out as she planned or imagined they would: the sweater is blue and she wanted red, the kids didn't say the right things when they got their presents, the soufflé fell, the camcorder ran out of tape. Her notions of Christmas perfection get in the way of her enjoying the day she has been given, as well as making everyone around her miserable.

How many holidays have been ruined because they didn't match someone's picture of how it was supposed to be? It's fine to plan for what you want from a holiday celebration, but be willing to be happy with what actually happens. Keep in mind that the good feelings you create together are the only things that matter.

What Would I Enjoy Doing?

One of the reasons the holidays are such energy- and money-depleting affairs is that we go around asking ourselves what we *should* do, rather than what we would like to do. We think we should buy everyone we know a present, send out an end-of-the-year letter to everyone in our address book, make cookies from scratch. . . . The list goes on and on.

Where do all the shoulds come from? Many of them come from family traditions that may or may not still be meaningful to us. Or our ideas of what is socially correct. What would happen if instead of shoulds this holiday season, we ask ourselves, "What would I really feel good about doing?" and then do only those things? Then our giving will come from our hearts, and the joy that is the true meaning of the season will enliven us and those around us.

This Is It

One of the wisest cartoons I have ever seen is a Gahan Wilson *New Yorker* cartoon. In it, two monks are sitting next to each other, meditating. One is young and seems confused; the other is old and serene. It's clear that the younger has asked the older a question. The old monk answers, "Nothing happens next. This is it."

I love that because for so long in my life, I thought that happiness was something to strive for, to work at, something that would come after I climbed the ladder, got the job, the relationship, the child. I kept waiting for happiness to grab hold of me, to announce itself as a permanent fixture once I did whatever I had to do to "make" it arrive. I thought if my husband would come home earlier, I would be happy. If I could make more money, I would be happy. *But this is it.* This life, the one we are experiencing right now, is the only life we have. And if we wait for all conditions to be perfect in order to be happy, chances are we will cheat ourselves out of our full measure of potential happiness. For happiness is here to be experienced right now, in this moment, no matter what else is going on in our lives.

This is it. Right now. Can you tap into the natural joy and happiness available in this moment just as it is?

Create a Great Family Gathering

Holidays can be great occasions for joyful togetherness, but often they are merely occasions for heartburn. Here are two ways to increase the happiness quotient from Dan Neuharth, Ph.D, author of *If You Had Controlling Parents:*

If you have meddling parents or other relatives, solicit their advice instead of waiting for them to butt in with their opinions: "Auntie, how do you think we should arrange the centerpiece?" "Dad, I'm having a problem at work. What do you think I should do?" They might even have something useful to suggest!

Bring out the photo albums and home videos: nothing helps more with family bonding than reminiscing over good times in the past. This will help take the attention off of your son's current haircut or how many pounds you put on.

Some other suggestions: Take a walk to cool off if the tension gets too high. Imagine you're watching a play, with all your family members the characters. This helps create emotional distance. Finally, if you really think being with your family will make you miserable, do something else instead.

Throw a Few Love Darts

"Love darts" were invented by my friend Sue Patton Thoele. They are silent blessings sent to people who are driving us crazy in some way, shape, or form. Rather than cursing the person silently or vociferously, Sue sends a good wish—"May you be happy," for example—which, if nothing else, reminds her to keep her heart open. "My favorite target," she says, "is a surly checkout person at the grocery store. I don't know how he feels about being pricked by a love dart, but I certainly feel better after sending one than I do if I grouse to myself about how rude he is."

Lighten your life a bit this holiday season by sending love darts today to everyone who in any way annoys or frustrates you.

Have a Winter Solstice Celebration

Today is the solstice, the shortest day of the year. Birds are often hungry at this time of year, when their food supplies are low or nonexistent. So hold a Winter Solstice celebration for the birds. It's particularly enjoyable if you have kids. But feel free to give it a try by yourself too!

First prepare the food—pine cones coated in peanut butter and bread cut out with cookie cutters for the birds (popcorn chains are good too) and whatever treats you might like for yourself. Tie up your bird goodies with yarn and hang from a tree. Light sparklers and sing songs, then retire inside for your part of the feast.

Banish the Winter Blues

I have a friend who was depressed for decades each winter. Then she discovered that she suffered from Seasonal Affective Disorder (SAD), a condition that affects 25 million Americans, particularly women. Reduced sunlight in the winter triggers brain chemistry changes that cause depression.

These are the symptoms: sadness that starts as the hours of sunlight get shorter (with my mother, it would come on in early fall); lower energy; food cravings; sleep disturbances; poor concentration; low sex drive. The great news is that it can be treated with light therapy: exposure to full-spectrum light bulbs or boxes during the winter. More than 80 percent of those suffering with SAD report at least some relief from light therapy, and recently researchers at the Oregon Health Sciences University in Portland have discovered that melatonin may help. Patients who received a .1 mg dose at 2, 4, and 6 P.M. found their symptoms eased, probably by an adjustment of the circadian rhythms. If you want to try this, researchers caution that melatonin can interfere with other drugs and can cause sleepiness, even in such a low dose. So if you suspect you might have SAD, read one of the good books on the subject and talk with your doctor.

Connect to the Divine

One of the difficulties of modern life is that we experience ourselves as separate from everyone and everything else. In their book *Contentment,* the great Jungian theorist Robert A. Johnson and coauthor Jerry M. Ruhl note that we "forget that there is a deeper layer of experience that we share with our whole culture and with all creation. This Jung called the collective unconscious—a source of wisdom, purpose and meaning." Because we are cut off from this source, we are filled with fear and insecurity. To be happy, say the authors, "our egos must circle around a steady, unmoving center, a source that is undisturbed by the whirl of life that goes on around it. . . . That's why Jung once wrote that the primary question people face today is, 'Are we related to something infinite or not?'"

When we tap into the infinite, we experience the deep happiness that comes from feeling that all is right with the world and our place in it. If you don't have a spiritual practice, consider cultivating one. And be guided by recent research that shows that people who consider themselves spiritual and regularly attend services are significantly more happy than those who don't call themselves spiritual, and those who are the most depressed are those who consider themselves spiritual but attend no services.

Do an Appreciation Ritual

I have written about this a lot because it is one of the most powerful things I have ever done for creating connection and happiness. You can do this anywhere, with anyone you know relatively well—family members, coworkers, kids. It's particularly great at holiday time. Here's how:

Sit in a circle. Choose one person as the focus and then everyone else, as the spirit moves them, speaks of why they appreciate that person. When everyone who wants to has spoken, go to another person until everyone has received appreciation. There are four rules:

1. Remarks must be positive (no sarcasm or backhanded compliments).

2. No cross-talk—no one else may interject anything while someone is speaking.

3. No one has to speak if he or she doesn't want to.

4. The object of praise may not say anything. The last rule is particularly hard. We tend to want to minimize or deflect compliments. But try just to take them in, as much as you can allow yourself.

Dedicate This Day

You can do this any day, but what better day than the occasion of the birth of Jesus Christ, the embodiment of love and compassion. Dedicate this Day is easy. All you do is send the positive feelings you are experiencing in this day to someone in need: for example, to those who have experienced childhood abuse, or to people who are alone.

Dedicate this Day is based on the principle that we are all, somehow, connected and that what happens to one part of the whole can affect the rest. Science is beginning to discover this (my favorite example is that bacteria in Petri dishes that are prayed for grow better than bacteria not prayed for), but we don't have to wait for proof to experience the joy that comes from silently sending our joy to others.

Give a Hug

Like so many other positive acts, it turns out that hugging boosts our immune systems. Plus it just plain feels good!

So hug someone today, perhaps a person who seems particularly in need.

Get an Energy Boost

Dragging around day after day? Maybe you need an energy boost to get moving and feel happier. The Herb Research Foundation suggests 360 mg daily of Siberian ginseng. It's great for increasing stamina (and might even keep you healthier—studies have shown that it cuts sick days as much as 40 percent). If you have trouble sleeping, try taking it before lunch so it can wear off by bedtime.

Be sure you buy a brand that has been standardized to 3–7 percent ginsenosides (some products have been found to have contaminants). A good bet is Ginsana. Avoid if you have high blood pressure, diabetes, cancer, or are taking blood thinners or antidepressants.

How Are You Growing?

*Happiness is neither virtue or pleasure, not this thing nor that, but
simply growth. We are happy when we are growing.*
—William Butler Yeats

I believe we are on Earth to grow our souls—to learn from
our woundedness, to become more loving, kind, compassionate, and to offer our unique gifts to the world. The
more we do this, the happier we'll be, regardless of our circumstances.

In what ways are you growing? Taking a risk to be
more yourself at work? Practicing dealing with anger in a
more healthy way? Right now, notice where you are growing. And if you respond nowhere, if you feel you're stagnating, reflect on where in your life you'd *like* to grow, and
begin.

Start Over

Recently I read a quote by a guy named Biker Steve. He said, "If your day isn't going well, start over. Even if it's a minute before midnight, start over. It's never too late."

What words of wisdom. It is never too late to start over, no matter what our circumstances. We can always begin again, right where we are. I think of an alcoholic I know who stopped drinking in his sixties and had ten years of sobriety before he passed on. Or a woman who went to college in her eighties. It's never to late to start over.

I was reminded of this recently by a friend who had been bemoaning the fact that when she turned forty, she had decided to dedicate the year to herself, to take stock and figure out what she wanted to do with the rest of her life. But then her father died and her two small children got sick again and again, and she came to the end of the year without finding the time. She was bemoaning the situation to her husband, who said to her, "But you can start now. It's not too late." And she did.

Where do you need to begin again? In a relationship? At work? With a child? Yourself? It's never too late.

What Do You Want More Of?

Really. What do you want more of in your life? More peace? More time off? More rest? More fun? More inner tranquility? Unless we identify what we truly want, we tend to be so caught up in daily life that we don't even think about what will make us truly happy. Today, ask yourself what you want more of in your life, and then live with the question all day: How can I have more _____ in my life? Just ask; don't worry about an answer. Don't squash the question with "but"s and "no"s—just let it reverberate in your consciousness.

When I ask myself that question today, the answer is, "More meaning." So I wonder how to bring more meaning into my life. As I sit with my wondering, more questions emerge—What is meaning to me? Does it involve other people or is it primarily internal? How would I know it if I had it? I don't try to answer any of these questions definitively. I just let them swirl around in my consciousness. As they do, an answer often pops up—usually sometime later, even weeks or months later—from somewhere unexpected: a book, a friend, a thought that occurs while driving. As Rilke says, "Be patient with the questions themselves."

Out with the Old, In with the New

New Year's Eve has always been a problem for me. I don't like staying up late, drinking too much, and ending up in a big crowd kissing everyone in sight. If that's your idea of happiness, then go for it. I prefer something quieter. I like to take the opportunity to focus on what I want to cultivate in the coming year. I do it by throwing the runes with my husband and writing down the messages so I can refer to them throughout the year.

But I also like a ritual done by Unity Church members, in which you write down what you are releasing on slips of paper—old habits of being, tired mental attitudes—and place them in a brass or ceramic bowl and burn them. Then you write down what you want to keep or take hold of—more peace and happiness, more compassion and generosity—and tuck those papers in your pocket.

You can do this with friends and family or alone. Or you can gather family members and talk about what you learned this past year. Choose a quality you all want to work on and dedicate the year to that quality: This year is the Year of Compassion. Or each select a quality to work on individually. Whatever you do, make it meaningful to you.

Index

To Our Readers

CONARI PRESS publishes books on topics ranging from spirituality, personal growth, and relationships to women's issues, parenting, and social issues. Our mission is to publish quality books that will make a difference in people's lives—how we feel about ourselves and how we relate to one another. We value integrity, compassion, and receptivity, both in the books we publish and in the way we do business.

As a member of the community, we sponsor the Random Acts of Kindness™ Foundation, the guiding force behind Random Acts of Kindness™ Week. We donate our damaged books to nonprofit organizations, dedicate a portion of our proceeds from certain books to charitable causes, and continually look for new ways to use natural resources as wisely as possible.

Our readers are our most important resource, and we value your input, suggestions, and ideas about what you would like to see published. Please feel free to contact us, to request our latest book catalog, or to be added to our mailing list.

2550 Ninth Street, Suite 101
Berkeley, California 94710-2551
800-685-9595   510-649-7175
fax: 510-649-7190   e-mail: conari@conari.com
http://www.conari.com